ALTERNATIVE MEDICINE, HEALTH AND WELLNESS

ALTERNATIVE MEDICINE

PERCEPTIONS, USES AND BENEFITS AND CLINICAL IMPLICATIONS

Alternative Medicine, Health and Wellness

Additional books in this series can be found on Nova's website under the Series tab.

Additional e-books in this series can be found on Nova's website under the eBooks tab.

ALTERNATIVE MEDICINE, HEALTH AND WELLNESS

ALTERNATIVE MEDICINE

PERCEPTIONS, USES AND BENEFITS AND CLINICAL IMPLICATIONS

E. PAUL CHERNIACK
AND
TASS HOLMES
EDITORS

NOVA BIOMEDICAL

New York

Library of Congress Cataloging-in-Publication Data

ISBN: 978-1-63484-826-8
Library of Congress Control Number: 20169333

Published by Nova Science Publishers, Inc. † New York

CONTENTS

PREFACE

Complementary and Alternative Medicine (CAM) today attracts significant attention through online health and consumer forums, professional CAM-practitioner associations and conferences, the recent growth in integrative biomedicine, and through the influence of advertisements and documentary presentations in mass media. A majority or large minority of consumers in developed countries regularly resort to professional CAM for supportive treatment for sickness in the form of chiropractic, osteopathic, prescribed dietary changes, acupuncture, massage, homeopathy, naturopathy and herbal medicine, and also use numerous associated lifestyle practices such as vegetarianism, nutritional supplementation, yoga and tai chi for self-treatment and to maintain general wellbeing. Many leading health insurance funds now provide generous rebates against out-of-pocket fees paid by consumers for private-sector CAM consultations. Furthermore, populations of developing countries continue to depend heavily on traditional herbal medicine and psycho-spiritual practices for their healing, on account of pharmaceutical treatments being often unaffordable or unavailable to them.

Despite CAM's prevalence, however, it continues to remain at the periphery of developed health systems, and usually attracts little government support and few subsidies. CAM is poorly defined in policy statements in many countries, although the NCCAM in USA and NHS in England are exceptions. Biomedical interests frequently cite a lack of scientific research evidence demonstrating CAM effectiveness as a primary reason for its general absence from policy and funding domains.

Nevertheless, contemporary research in CAM now represents an extremely broad and rapidly expanding field, with studies ranging from random controlled trials and demographic consumer studies, to anthropological representations of “traditional medicine” and explanations of the distinctive holistic CAM healing paradigms. This volume provides a helpful synthesis of recent research by diverse international contributors from several sub-fields of the health and research endeavor.

Chapters of the book include literature reviews (such as study findings about the benefits of CAM for elderly persons and of laughter therapy, from the USA, and herbal treatments for pain, in Mauritius), and original studies (poor CAM consumers in Australia, the location of naturopaths’ practice in Canada, and the use of mindfulness meditation among nursing students in Scotland). Study findings presented here are enjoyable in their diversity, and add to contemporary literature both by presenting common perceptions about CAM, by engaging in discussion of its prevalence and popularity in diverse contexts, and the contentious topic of placebo effect and questions as to how to prove effectiveness for alternative healing methods, further reviewing some potential clinical benefits.

Chapter 1- Ten years ago, the author edited a textbook on the use of alternative medicine by the elderly. The purpose of the present chapter is to briefly highlight significant improvements in our understanding of the use of alternative medicine by this growing segment of the world’s population, by summarizing recent published literature on this topic. An opening section describes the prevalence and rationale for use of complementary and alternative medicine (CAM), drawn from epidemiological studies, followed by an overview of recent research on CAM therapies, for specific mental and physical conditions.

Chapter 2 - Complementary and alternative medicine (CAM) is in widespread use among Australians. This chapter, diverging from demographic studies and professional naturopathic literature, presents the findings of an anthropological study in a small Victoria-state Australian rural community, designated ‘Sephirah’. It explores CAM use by poorer residents of local townships, the provision of professional CAM to low-income rural people by practitioners, and the cultural and spiritual meanings and significance CAM held for research participants.

The study’s findings suggest both self-prescribed and professionally-provided CAM are frequently resorted to by ‘inner-rural’ dwelling Australians, who often harbour alternative worldviews, linking CAM use for health maintenance to nature-oriented, non-mainstream political and spiritual beliefs.

Retaining a more-or-less marginal status relative to biomedicine, CAM nevertheless represents a health agency or activist position for many consumers who lack faith in the modernist biomedical approach, thereby contributing both to wellbeing and enhanced social-cultural identity. The sense of an 'inherent' CAM-linked agency is a refreshing discovery of the research.

Chapter 3 - With the use of an Ontario-wide dataset of naturopathic doctor (ND) office locations and a survey from patients of five naturopaths in the communities of Waterloo and Greater Sudbury, it is determined that NDs (like chiropractors and dentists) are attracted to the vicinity of high visibility areas, although somewhat paradoxically, the majority of patients are not concerned with their ND's location. High visibility areas include those on, within or near main roads, high traffic land use and high population density neighborhoods. In aggregate, the patients consider quality of service and reputation to be much more important than distance to an ND's office. It is speculated that the value of a high visibility location to a naturopath may vary by the ND's length of time in business, the possibility of appealing to less affluent populations and likely agglomeration economies advantages (that is, the benefits of clustering within a given space).

Chapter 4 - Nursing students are exposed to stress when they undertake clinical placements and stress may be associated with increasing attrition rates in nursing undergraduate courses. Mindfulness meditation training has previously been shown to reduce stress in registered nurses. This chapter describes a mixed methods feasibility study which examined the usefulness and effectiveness of mindfulness meditation in improving situational stress-response resilience in nursing students. The chapter concludes by identifying recommendations for future mindfulness meditation research methodologies. Recommendations are also made for nursing undergraduate curriculum and undergraduate nursing student support services development.

Chapter 5 - Complementary and alternative medicine (CAM) approaches are growing in popularity for the treatment of psychological conditions, particularly to supplement pharmaceutical and psychotherapeutic therapies. There is a need for better communication between the patient, physician, and alternative practitioners, as well as for physicians and pharmacists to become more informed to be able to best benefit patients choosing to employ these options and to prevent interaction effects.

Chapter 6 - Pain essentially is a mere sensation which acts as herald of danger to the body, nonetheless once pain transcends the prognosis stage, it becomes no less than an ordeal resulting in repercussions including anxiety, depression, sleep disturbances, amongst others on patients' daily life. Such is the intricacy of pain that the contribution of conventional medicine in its relief despite conspicuous yet remains below par as far as management of arthritis pain, diabetic neuropathy, cancer pain, fibromyalgia, and other related conditions are concerned wherein substantial pain is endured by patients. Accordingly, due to particular constraints of mainstream medicine, there has been the resurgence and extensive use of alternative medicine in current years endorsed by ever mounting evidence of its efficacy. The success of alternative medicine has been irrefutable and momentous in alleviating chronic pain conditions. This chapter attempts to overview pain and its physiology, the role of inflammation in pain perception, the classification of pain, pain assessment tools, common chronic pain conditions, widespread alternative therapies used for pain management and specific challenges of alternative medicine.

Chapter 7 - Laughter therapy refers to a treatment modality in which a facilitator induces or trains patients to laugh (with or without humor) to obtain physiologic or psychological benefit. Related, but not synonymous modalities include humor therapy, which specifically uses humor as a treatment to improve the health of patients which may not necessarily involve laughter, and laughter yoga, a type of exercise developed by an Indian physician in which a therapist leads patients to clap, chant stretch, breathe, and laugh without the inducement of humor. All of these modalities may confer related health benefits, though laughter and humor therapy have not been studied as intensively as laughter yoga.

PART ONE: USERS

In: Alternative Medicine ISBN: 978-1-63484-826-8
Editors: E. P. Cherniack and T. Holmes © 2016 Nova Science Publishers, Inc.

Chapter 1

UPDATE ON THE USE OF ALTERNATIVE MEDICINE BY THE ELDERLY

E. Paul Cherniack
Geriatrics and Extended Care Service and Geriatric Research, Education, and Clinical Center (GRECC) of the Miami Veterans Affairs Medical Center, and the Division of Geriatrics and Palliative Medicine, University of Miami Miller School of Medicine, Miami FL, US

ABSTRACT

Ten years ago, I edited a textbook on the use of alternative medicine by the elderly [1]. The purpose of the present chapter is to briefly highlight significant improvements in our understanding of the use of alternative medicine by this growing segment of the world's population, by summarizing recent published literature on this topic. An opening section describes the prevalence and rationale for use of complementary and alternative medicine (CAM), drawn from epidemiological studies, followed by an overview of recent research on CAM therapies, for specific mental and physical conditions.

EPIDEMIOLOGIC STUDIES

While users of CAM have often been described as predominately young and female, many investigations continue to document the persistent use of

CAM by older individuals. Specific correlates of CAM use have been inconsistent, probably due to demographic differences and attitudes toward CAM uses in different study populations. In a randomized cross-sectional survey from Minnesota of 1200 independently-living participants age 65 or over, 62.9% used CAM [2]. Supplements (44.3%) and prayer or spiritual rituals (29.7%) were the most commonly employed means. Older persons most frequently utilized CAM to treat arthritis and other pain, although they were more concerned with "maintaining health" (73.7%) than "treating a health condition" (59.6%). Neither gender was more likely to use CAM. Another investigation of 8587 independently-living individuals in Australia, by contrast, found men were more commonly CAM users than women (O.R. 1.79; 95% C.I. 0.94-2.34) [3]. Women who utilized CAM described themselves as in poorer health and in pain, in contrast to men. In a third survey, drawn from a convenience sample of 338 predominantly male attendees of an urban US Veterans Administration hospital clinic in Florida, mean age 77.5, gender and ethnicity strongly influenced CAM use [4]. Far more women (66%) used CAM than men (29%), and Hispanics (64%) were more likely to utilize CAM than blacks (46%) or whites (19%).

As CAM may be used for symptomatic self-management, several efforts specifically examined the use of CAM as self-help treatment. Based on data collected from elderly people in several rural US counties, 24.2% of elders used home remedies, 21.7% used herbal treatments, and 58.7% employed prayer to treat their symptoms [5]. The most commonly used herbal treatments were echinacea, garlic, and ginkgo biloba, and 31.7 combined herbal and conventional therapies [6].

Use of CAM as adjunctive therapies to treat specific illnesses has provided a focus of other investigations. Relatively few elderly cancer patients about to undergo chemotherapy, participating in a US multi-center trial of 545 people, consumed CAM (17%) [7]. One might speculate that such individuals may be more motivated to rely on conventional medicine than CAM. By comparison, twenty-seven women, ages 65 to 93, who employed CAM to treat their arthritis, in a qualitative analysis, believed their disease was incurable, that conventional medicine did not provide a sufficient range of options to treat their symptoms, and that CAM might offer an effective palliative treatment for them [8].

The utilization of specific CAM modalities by older individuals, such as folk medicine, has also been studied. For example, twenty-two percent of elderly individuals in China use Tai Chi [9]. However, a review of 25 studies concerned with the consumption of folk medicine by the elderly failed to find specific demographic characteristics that correlated with folk medicine utilization [10]. Participants of these investigations relied on a diverse group of methods, that often stemmed from the older persons' specific cultural backgrounds. Many of the research subjects did not notify conventional practitioners about their folk medicine use.

A potentially important consideration in the elderly concerns the provision of CAM to institutionalized residents. A systematic review identified only five published studies considering this topic, none of which specified the prevalence of CAM use among the residents [11]. In a survey of Chinese medicine use, consumers reported that institutional staff members sometimes lacked information about CAM, and also desired to avoid any potential medico-legal problems they believed could ensue from use of CAM [12].

Some studies considered the reasons why older persons choose to use CAM. Numerous hypotheses proposed as explanations for CAM utilization by the elderly including a desire for control over health care, acknowledgement that there are illnesses for which conventional medicine has no good answers, and belief in the efficacy of CAM [13]. Recent surveys emphasize the commonality of the first of these explanations, that is, a desire of elderly patients to maintain control over their healthcare decisions. Participants in a focus group discussing CAM use described dissatisfaction with strictly pharmaceutical approaches to healthcare, including the possible risk of adverse events, and harbored a belief that conventional medicine continues to view aging as a process of inevitable decline in health, contrary to their own personal views, and a that CAM offers a means of self-empowerment [14]. Another focus group, comprised of elderly Australian women, similarly expressed views of self-empowerment, and a desire to circumvent problems associated with a conventional medical approach [15]. Volition for self-empowerment and control was also associated with use of CAM in a cross-sectional survey of 296 lung cancer patients attending a university oncology clinic [16]. Nevertheless, among rural elderly in the US, disbelief in the efficacy of conventional medication or belief in one's own behavior as a prime determinant of health were not generally associated with CAM use [17].

Other surveys have described geographic variations in CAM use by older persons. In an investigation of 400 subjects in Germany, living in a variety of settings, most believed CAM improved their symptoms, but were unable to determine if chosen modalities created adverse reactions [18]. In another survey of 5830 older subjects, gleaned from elderly insurance records in Germany, CAM consumers most commonly used CAM in conjunction with conventional treatments [19, 20]. Men preferred physical modalities (e.g., acupuncture) to ingested treatments. Conversely, women opted for herbal therapy more often than men, but most frequently preferred acupuncture (21%) and homeopathy (21%), among all the CAM modalities used.

CAM utilization has been investigated in several studies from Jordan. Among a sample of 143 outpatients with chronic illnesses, a pharmacist interviewed subjects and recorded herbal treatments they consumed. The most common were *Hibiscus sabdariffa L.* (22.6%), ginger (15.1%), and olive leaves and olive oil (20.7% combined) [21]. Similar investigations were conducted in the Jordanian capital of 1000 attendees of the national diabetic treatment institutes, and a further 50 subjects selected at random from those visiting a cancer center [22, 23]. Diabetics most frequently consumed green tea (20.5%), *Pimpinella anisum L.* (19.9%), ginger (18.7%), and chamomile (18.1%). Sixty-nine percent took these substances for symptomatic relief. One-third of the group of the cancer patients used herbal remedies, seventy-three percent in liquid form. Finally, a number of studies delineated differences in the ways CAM is employed in certain geographic settings. For example, more than half of a sample of 71 diabetics in rural USA engaged in prayer (57%) or utilized dietary forms of CAM (13%) [24].

Studies on Specific CAM Modalities

CAM to treat mental health issues: Mind-body method, stress-reduction technique, yoga, meditation, relaxation, music listening, Tai Chi, exercise, massage and herbal medicines

Considerable research has explored the use of CAM to treat mental health. Some investigations delineated demographic characteristics of CAM consumers who employ CAM specifically for mental health concerns. A survey of older persons who utilized mind-body techniques to treat depression showed racial but not educational differences [25]. In this survey, black Americans were more likely to opt for 'mind-body techniques', as were women and younger participants. Among individuals sampled in the (US) National Health Interview Survey, younger women, blacks, and Asians more frequently chose mind-body medicine [26].

Many recent studies have piloted non-pharmacological interventions to treat mental health. In one prospective investigation, 100 people at least 65 years of age took part in activities to reduce stress, including meditation and yoga, before and after which two stress-related cytokine levels were measured, insulin-like growth-related factor-1 (IGF-1), and interleukin-6 (IL-6) [27].

Participants exhibited significantly lowered IGF-1 concentrations after participation, although IL-6 concentrations were not significantly affected by the intervention. In another study, twenty people, all over 55 years, who participated in either yoga or meditation, had neuropsychological testing [28]. Those individuals active in yoga displayed improved attention scores. A further thirteen elderly women with osteoarthritis undertook one hour and fifteen minute yoga classes once a week for two months, to improve their sleep [29]. These subjects noted gains across several measures of sleep function, including efficiency, sleep onset latency, and insomnia-free nights.

In a nursing home-based intervention, 50 elderly residents, aged at least 55, were randomized to participate in a 30 minute weekly music listening session or a rest session [30]. Those in the treatment group could sample selections of one of four types of music and choose what they preferred to listen to. The mean Geriatric Depression Scale score at the onset of the experiment was 4.23 in the control and 4.17 in the music group. After two months, music listeners reduced their mean scores to 1.38 ($p = 0.006$ change from baseline) whereas those who merely rested had an unchanged mean score.

A further trial that employed music and rest studied 93 older persons living outside of institutions, with a mean age of 70, who listened to a CD that provided instruction in both guided imagery and relaxation. These research subjects learned to use visual imagery to imagine themselves performing various physical activities, and undertook sequential tensing and relaxing of muscle groups and the performance of deep breathing exercises (for relaxation), followed by a music listening session in which they listened to songs of their choice [31]. A control group heard relaxation instructions and music only. Study subjects listened to the CD twice a week for six weeks, for at least 10 minutes per session. At the onset and completion of the experiment, participants answered questionnaires about exercise participation and subjective attitudes toward exercise. Those who took part in the guided imagery reported they performed significantly more exercise than those in the control group.

In a small uncontrolled investigation, a massage therapist provided daily ten minute foot massage to seventeen nursing home residents with dementia, for two weeks [32]. At the end of the study, individuals who had received massage obtained significantly lower scores (respectively, 22% reduction and 16% reduction on scales rating agitation and memory impairment, the Cohen-Mansfield Agitation Inventory, and the Revised Memory and Behavior

Problems Checklist). These benefits persisted for two weeks after conclusion of the treatments.

Several trials have studied the effect of Tai Chi to address mental health issues. Sixty-two nursing home residents in Iran, at least sixty years of age, undertook Tai Chi exercise for 20 to 25 minutes, three times a week for three months, or no exercise [33]. Participants exercising experienced significant improvement on the Pittsburgh Sleep Quality Index at the close of the intervention.

In another trial, 112 depressed elderly persons, aged at least a 60, who previously experienced a response to the antidepressant escitalopram either underwent weekly two-hour Tai Chi sessions, or received health education for the same length of time [34]. The subjects who trained in performing Tai Chi exercises showed a significantly better rating on the Hamilton Depression Rating Score than those who were not trained (5.1 vs. 6.7, $p = 0.001$). A metaanalysis concluded that Tai Chi improved sleep, as measured by the Pittsburgh Sleep Quality Index [35]. In another study, eighty-three people without depression, between the ages 59 and 86, performed four months of Tai Chi, or had health education, however those learning Tai Chi did not found experience any greater decrease in depressive symptoms [36].

Another Oriental exercise regimen was piloted, to improve sleep in older individuals [37]. Fifty-five community-dwelling Taiwanese individuals, at least 60 years old, participated in a Chinese exercise called Baduanjin, featuring maneuvers that are neither taxing, rapid, or difficult to learn. The subjects watched a video, had one week of instruction, and were urged to practice half an hour per day, three times a week for three months, and to log their efforts. A control group did no exercise. The elderly persons who exercised reported better sleep efficiency, quality, duration, and less latency.

Other studies have explored the effects of herbal treatments on mental health. A minority of elderly individuals have been found to self-medicate with plant remedies in addition to conventional treatments, such as St. John's Wort and serotonergic medications, to alleviate depressive symptoms [38].

In one investigation, twenty-eight older individuals (at least age 75) had cognitive testing, and then consumed 0.75-6gm of rosemary powder mixed with tomato juice after which they repeated testing at several intervals over a six hour assessment period [39]. On one measure of memory speed, subjects realized a significantly improved score at the 0.75gm dose, but a worse score at the highest dose. There were further significant but non-dose dependent differences on tests of attention and memory.

A more widely used herbal medicine has been gingko biloba. However, in two large studies over six years, in several thousand subjects, gingko failed both to prevent dementia and to reduce the rate of cognitive decline in normal elderly subjects [40, 41].

CAM for physical health: Tai Chi, yoga, massage, acupuncture, Traditional Chinese Medicine, dance and video games

Tai Chi

Much research has focused on using CAM to improve physical health of the elderly, and a major focus of this body of research has again been Tai Chi. In one intervention, for instance, 26 participants, with a mean age of 61.5, obtained weekly advice on diet over a four month period, with or without participation in a 45 minute Tai Chi class three times per week [42]. There were no differences in weight loss between the intervention and control groups, but those who undertook Tai Chi made greater improvements in lipid-lowering dietary choices. In another trial, Tai Chi was employed to correct the balance of visually-impaired older persons. Forty subjects with low vision attended Tai Chi classes lasting 90 minutes, three times a week for four months, or, in a control group, received instruction on playing a musical instrument. Tai Chi-trained individuals experienced significant benefits in tests of sensory proprioception, the Sensory Organization Test and the passive knee joint repositioning test [43]. A further, twenty elderly persons who performed Tai Chi for 3 months, one hour per session, three times a week, achieved significant gains in soleus muscle strength [44]. Forty community-dwelling older individuals between the ages of 60 and 80, complaining of "dizziness", participated in a 45 minute bi-weekly Tai Chi class for two and half months, or a control conventional exercise program [45]. At completion of the program, those who undertook Tai Chi had significantly better results on an eight-foot Up and Go Test (in which subjects were required arise from a chair, walk eight feet, and return), and other parameters measured by a computerized balance assessment platform. For another twenty-eight older individuals, training in Tai Chi enhanced their ability to stand on one leg and step down from a platform [46].

Not all trials have confirmed a positive effect of Tai Chi on balance in the elderly. In a further study, 34 non-institutionalized older persons were trained in hour-long Tai Chi classes three times a week for three months, but no improvement to postural stability was observed [44]. A larger trial contrasted the effects of Tai Chi with conventional therapy in 152 subjects aged 65, who attended a Canadian day hospital. The participants undertook 15 weeks of 4.5 hours a week of Tai Chi, or took part in a control program of other physical therapy. Both groups had fewer falls at the end of the intervention, although the Tai Chi group was more successful (RR = 0.74; 95% CI = 0.56-0.98) [47]. Both groups also showed improved measurements in parameters of gait and balance, other than number of falls. Nevertheless, no statistical differences between the groups existed, except for a higher rating of self-efficacy by the Tai Chi group [47]. Despite a number of studies affirming benefits of Tai Chi practice for improving balance and helping prevent falls, a Cochrane review of trials of various interventions to lower the incidence of falls noted the effect of Tai Chi to be of "borderline" significance [48].

Yoga, Dance, Video Games and Massage Therapy

In addition to its benefits on mental health, yoga has been studied for potential improvements to physical performance. In one small trial, eight subjects whose mean age was 84, participated in two months of yoga, for an hour and forty minutes, twice weekly [49]. Before and after the intervention they received balance assessment using the Berg Balance Scale, the Timed Up and Go Test, and a gait speed measurement. These elderly subjects obtained significant benefits from yoga, both in their balance evaluation, and in gait speed. Another fifty-four community-living Australians, with a mean age 68, undertook 3 months of an hourly yoga program two times a week. A control group was given a copy of a falls prevention guide. Those receiving yoga observed an improvement in standing balance [50]. A review and metaanalysis of the results of eighteen small studies on the effects of yoga noted mild physical benefits [51].

Dancing, like yoga, is a physical CAM modality that has been piloted in investigations for its potential to enhance physical performance. In one dance study, twenty-eight elderly subjects were enrolled in a two-month program of salsa dancing, or a control group without dancing [52]. Salsa participants demonstrated augmented stride length and velocity, but did not increase power in leg extensors or decrease gait variability. In another trial, twenty-seven individuals who received eighteen 45-minute dance lessons, performing steps based on ballet and jazz, failed to improve either balance or mobility [53].

Video games have also been used similarly to enhance mobility. Twenty-eight healthy elderly Danish study subjects living in the community, with a mean age of 75, received two and a half months of physiotherapy to improve strength and balance, augmented by biofeedback training using a Nintendo Wii [54]. A control group received conventional physiotherapy treatment and new shoe insoles. Subjects taking part in Wii training obtained an 18% better measure of maximal voluntary contraction strength and a quicker Timed Up and Go Test, although their overall balance was not improved.

Massage therapy is another common CAM modality offering potential physical and mental health benefits. In a survey, 144 participants who received massage treatments during the past 12 months were compared to those who had not [55]. Massage recipients perceived they had fewer physical and emotional health problems than non-recipients. In a further study, 60 people, aged at least 60, with chronic pain, who obtained massage treatments reported significantly less pain, less disability, a higher energy level, and a better emotional state compared to non-recipients [56].

Acupuncture, Chinese Medicine, Mindfulness Meditation and Integrative Medicine

Acupuncture is another well-studied treatment with application for older individuals. An investigation of thirty-two people aged 61-81, with low back pain, randomized subjects to obtain acupuncture, transcutaneous electrical nerve stimulation (TENS), or both, or a topical analgesic cream with methylsalicylic acid [57]. Those treated with a combination of acupuncture and TENS experienced better pain control ($p < 0.008$) and quality of life ($p < 0.008$) than recipients of individual modalities. In a preceding trial of thirty-two individuals, also aged 61 to 81, who had knee osteoarthritis, recipients of the combination therapy perceived less pain from their condition ($p = 0.039$) and better knee function ($p = 0.008$) [58]. In yet another thirty subjects of similar ages, true acupuncture proved superior to sham acupuncture in perceived pain relief [59].

In an intervention based on Chinese medicine, 59 community-dwelling older residents of Hong Kong with knee osteoarthritis received localized massages with ginger and orange oil, an olive oil control, or conventional analgesic treatment [60]. Therapists provided subjects with six half-hour massages, during a treatment period of two to three weeks. Recipients of ginger and orange oil therapy reported significantly reduced knee pain and stiffness.

One trial utilized Chinese medicine to treat pain associated with herpes zoster [61]. Thirty-two subjects who were identified as having herpes zoster obtained a Chinese medical treatment comprising a combination of application of Chinese herbal formula, acupuncture, cupping (after injection of an anesthetic, bleeding was created at a spot with a lancet, and a suction cup applied to induce a vacuum), and meditation education (subjects listened to an instruction tape). A control group of 27 subjects was put on a wait list for the treatment. The mean age of subjects was 69.8 years. Three weeks after both groups completed the randomization phase, those in the treatment group rated their mean pain on a 10 point Likert scale (0-10, 10 = most pain) as 2.3, whereas the control group scored their mean pain at 7.5 ($p = 0.05$). The improvement in pain control persisted for over two months post-treatment.

Another method of CAM therapy, mindfulness meditation, has been piloted as an intervention to lower blood pressure in elderly persons [62]. Twenty individuals, at least 62 years old, received two months of an intervention, comprising hour and a half meditation lessons each week or participation in a social support group. Meditators lowered their systolic blood pressure by a mean 21.9 points ($p = 0.02$) and diastolic by 16.7 points ($p = 0.003$) compared to the control group.

Finally, rather than examining potential benefits of an individual CAM treatment, one pilot study assessed the feasibility of an entire program of "integrative medicine" [63]. In this investigation, twenty-nine elderly residents of shared apartment communities, who were at least 70 years old, attended a year-long program in which they took part in an hour-long exercise program once weekly, and received treatment from nurses trained by a naturopath, including naturopathic bandaging techniques, herbal topical oils and teas, dietary juice supplementation, and homeopathic remedies. A similar control group received conventional medical care, including physiotherapy. However, significant differences between the groups for measures of in activities of daily living, quality of life, or depression indices were not observed.

Can CAM Treatment Be Harmful to the Elderly?

Potential harms of CAM treatment in the elderly have not been well documented. In theory, taking extra supplements might reduce adherence to conventional medication in a population already plagued by polypharmacy

[64]. Among 180 hypertensive subjects over 65 who participated in a telephone survey, blacks, but not whites who used CAM were less likely to adhere to their antihypertensive medication regimens (O.R. = 1.56; 95% CI 1.14-2.15) [65]. On the other hand, in a sample of US veterans in Florida, there was no association between CAM use and adherence to conventional medication [66]. Differences in attitudes about CAM and conventional medical therapy in different populations studied might explain conflicting results. One recent study noted skepticism about conventional medicine was prevalent in a rural population, that might have been denied access to conventional medicine, however this attitude was not associated with CAM use [67].

Conclusion

Despite decades of research, there is a shortage of conclusive evidence of benefits of CAM modalities for older populations. This is unfortunate, when many CAM modalities, including Tai Chi and meditation, do not require older health consumers to have to remember to take yet another substance, adding to the toxicity and side-effect risks they face from polypharmacy, with this age group being especially vulnerable [68]. In select populations of older individuals who have sufficient cognitive understanding, and financial resources, and presuming a ready availability of CAM and CAM providers, certain non-medical modalities, such as Tai Chi, yoga, or meditation, might be considered low-risk adjunctive therapies, with additional potential subjective benefit for many users.

References

[1] Cherniack, EP. Alternative Medicine for the Elderly. Berlin: Springer, 2003.

[2] Cheung, CK; Wyman, JF; Halcon, LL. Use of complementary and alternative therapies in community-dwelling older adults. *J Altern Complement Med.*, 2007, 13, 997-1006.

[3] McLaughlin, D; Adams, J; Sibbritt, D; Lui, CW. Sex differences in the use of complementary and alternative medicine in older men and women. *Australas J Ageing.*, 2012, 31, 78-82.

[4] Cherniack, EP; Ceron-Fuentes, J; Florez, H; Sandals, L; Rodriguez, O; Palacios, JC. Influence of race and ethnicity on alternative medicine as a self-treatment preference for common medical conditions in a population of multi-ethnic urban elderly. *Complement Ther Clin Pract.*, 2008, 14, 116-123.

[5] Arcury, TA; Grzywacz, JG; Neiberg, RH; et al. Older adults' self-management of daily symptoms: complementary therapies, self-care, and medical care. *Journal of Aging and Health.*, 2012, 24, 569-597.

[6] Arcury, TA; Grzywacz, JG; Bell, RA; Neiberg, RH; Lang, W; Quandt, SA. Herbal remedy use as health self-management among older adults. *J Gerontol B Psychol Sci Soc Sci.*, 2007, 62, S142-149.

[7] Maggiore, RJ; Gross, CP; Togawa, K; et al. Use of complementary medications among older adults with cancer. *Cancer.*, 2012, 118, 4815-4823.

[8] Cheung, C. Complementary/alternative therapy use in older women with arthritis. *Res Gerontol Nurs.*, 2012, 5, 275-283.

[9] Birdee, GS; Cai, H; Xiang, YB; et al. T'ai chi as exercise among middle-aged and elderly Chinese in urban China. *J Altern Complement Med.*, 2013, 19, 550-557.

[10] Sackett, K; Carter, M; Stanton, M. Elders' use of folk medicine and complementary and alternative therapies: an integrative review with implications for case managers. *Prof Case Manag.*, 2014, 19, 113-123, quiz 124-115.

[11] Bauer, M; Rayner, JA. Use of complementary and alternative medicine in residential aged care. *J Altern Complement Med.*, 2012, 18, 989-993.

[12] Wong, EL; Lam, JK; Griffiths, S; Chung, V; Yeoh, EK. Chinese medicine: its role and application in the institutionalised older people. *J Clin Nurs.*, 2010, 19, 1084-1093.

[13] Furnham, A. Why do the elderly use complementary and alternative medicine. In: Cherniack P, Cherniack, N, editor. Alternative Medicine for the Elderly. Berlin: Springer, 2003, 9-25.

[14] Fries, CJ. Older adults' use of complementary and alternative medical therapies to resist biomedicalization of aging. *J Aging Stud.*, 2014, 28, 1-10.

[15] McLaughlin, D; Lui, CW; Adams, J. Complementary and alternative medicine use among older Australian women--a qualitative analysis. *BMC Complement Altern Med.*, 2012, 12, 34.

[16] Bauml, J; Langer, CJ; Evans, T; Garland, SN; Desai, K; Mao, JJ. Does perceived control predict Complementary and Alternative Medicine

(CAM) use among patients with lung cancer? A cross-sectional survey. *Supportive Care in Cancer.*, 2014.

[17] Bell, RA; Grzywacz, JG; Quandt, SA; et al. Medical skepticism and complementary therapy use among older rural African-Americans and Whites. *J Health Care Poor Underserved.*, 2013, 24, 777-787.

[18] Schnabel, K; Binting, S; Witt, CM; Teut, M. Use of complementary and alternative medicine by older adults - a cross-sectional survey. *BMC Geriatr.*, 2014, 14, 38.

[19] Bussing, A; Ostermann, T; Heusser, P; Matthiessen, PF. Usage of complementary and alternative medicine interventions by German older adults. *J Altern Complement Med.*, 2011, 17, 487-489.

[20] Bussing, A; Ostermann, T; Heusser, P; Matthiessen, PF. Usage of alternative medical systems, acupuncture, homeopathy and anthroposophic medicine, by older German adults. *Zhong Xi Yi Jie He Xue Bao.*, 2011, 9, 847-856.

[21] Wazaify, M; Alawwa, I; Yasein, N; Al-Saleh, A; Afifi, FU. Complementary and alternative medicine (CAM) use among Jordanian patients with chronic diseases. *Complement Ther Clin Pract.*, 2013, 19, 153-157.

[22] Wazaify, M; Afifi, FU; El-Khateeb, M; Ajlouni, K. Complementary and alternative medicine use among Jordanian patients with diabetes. *Complement Ther Clin Pract.*, 2011, 17, 71-75.

[23] Afifi, FU; Wazaify, M; Jabr, M; Treish, E. The use of herbal preparations as complementary and alternative medicine (CAM) in a sample of patients with cancer in Jordan. *Complement Ther Clin Pract.*, 2010, 16, 208-212.

[24] Bell, RA; Quandt, SA; Grzywacz, JG; et al. Patterns of Complementary Therapy Use for Symptom Management for Older Rural Adults with Diabetes. *J Evid Based Complementary Altern Med.*, 2013, 18.

[25] Morano, C; Giunta, N; Parikh, NS; Panuska, S; Fahs, MC; Gallo, WT. Mind-body techniques, race-ethnicity, and depression among urban senior center participants. *Health and Social Work.*, 2013, 38, 167-172.

[26] Prasad, K; Ziegenfuss, JY; Cha, SS; Sood, A; Tilburt, JC. Characteristics of exclusive users of mind-body medicine vs. other alternative medicine approaches in the United States. Explore (NY)., 2013, 9, 219-225.

[27] Gallegos, AM; Hoerger, M; Talbot, NL; et al. Toward identifying the effects of the specific components of Mindfulness-Based Stress Reduction on biologic and emotional outcomes among older adults. *J Altern Complement Med.*, 2013, 19, 787-792.

[28] Prakash, R; Rastogi, P; Dubey, I; Abhishek, P; Chaudhury, S; Small, BJ. Long-term concentrative meditation and cognitive performance among older adults. *Neuropsychol Dev Cogn B Aging Neuropsychol Cogn.*, 2012, 19, 479-494.

[29] Taibi, DM; Vitiello, MV. A pilot study of gentle yoga for sleep disturbance in women with osteoarthritis. *Sleep Med.*, 2011, 12, 512-517.

[30] Chan, MF; Wong, ZY; Onishi, H; Thayala, NV. Effects of music on depression in older people: a randomised controlled trial. *J Clin Nurs.*, 2012, 21, 776-783.

[31] Kim, BH; Newton, RA; Sachs, ML; Giacobbi, PR; Glutting, JJ. The effect of guided relaxation and exercise imagery on self-reported leisure-time exercise behaviors in older adults. *J Aging Phys Act.*, 2011, 19, 137-146.

[32] Moyle, W; Johnston, AN; O'Dwyer, ST. Exploring the effect of foot massage on agitated behaviours in older people with dementia: a pilot study. *Australas J Ageing.*, 2011, 30, 159-161.

[33] Hosseini, H; Esfirizi, MF; Marandi, SM; Rezaei, A. The effect of Ti Chi exercise on the sleep quality of the elderly residents in Isfahan, Sadeghieh elderly home. *Iran J Nurs Midwifery Res.*, 2011, 16, 55-60.

[34] Lavretsky, H; Alstein, LL; Olmstead, RE; et al. Complementary use of tai chi chih augments escitalopram treatment of geriatric depression: a randomized controlled trial. *Am J Geriatr Psychiatry.*, 2011, 19, 839-850.

[35] Du, S; Dong, J; Zhang, H; et al. Taichi exercise for self-rated sleep quality in older people: A systematic review and meta-analysis. *International Journal of Nursing Studies.*, 2014.

[36] Irwin, MR; Olmstead, R. Mitigating cellular inflammation in older adults: a randomized controlled trial of Tai Chi Chih. *Am J Geriatr Psychiatry.*, 2012, 20, 764-772.

[37] Chen, MC; Liu, HE; Huang, HY; Chiou, AF. The effect of a simple traditional exercise programme (Baduanjin exercise) on sleep quality of older adults: a randomized controlled trial. *International Journal of Nursing Studies.*, 2012, 49, 265-273.

[38] Rahman, SZ; Basilakis, J; Rahmadi, A; et al. Use of serotonergic antidepressants and St John's wort in older Australians: a population-based cohort study. *Australas Psychiatry.*, 2013, 21, 262-266.

[39] Pengelly, A; Snow, J; Mills, SY; Scholey, A; Wesnes, K; Butler, LR. Short-term study on the effects of rosemary on cognitive function in an elderly population. *J Med Food.*, 2012, 15, 10-17.

[40] DeKosky, ST; Williamson, JD; Fitzpatrick, AL; et al. Ginkgo biloba for prevention of dementia: a randomized controlled trial. *JAMA.*, 2008, 300, 2253-2262.

[41] Snitz, BE; O'Meara, ES; Carlson, MC; et al. Ginkgo biloba for preventing cognitive decline in older adults: a randomized trial. *JAMA.*, 2009, 302, 2663-2670.

[42] Beebe, N; Magnanti, S; Katkowski, L; et al. Effects of the addition of t'ai chi to a dietary weight loss program on lipoprotein atherogenicity in obese older women. *J Altern Complement Med.*, 2013, 19, 759-766.

[43] Chen, EW; Fu, AS; Chan, KM; Tsang, WW. The effects of Tai Chi on the balance control of elderly persons with visual impairment: a randomised clinical trial. *Age Ageing.*, 2012, 41, 254-259.

[44] Chen, YS; Zhou, S; Cartwright, C. Effect of 12 weeks of Tai Chi training on soleus Hoffmann reflex and control of static posture in older adults. *Arch Phys Med Rehabil.*, 2011, 92, 886-891.

[45] Maciaszek, J; Osinski, W. Effect of Tai Chi on body balance: randomized controlled trial in elderly men with dizziness. *Am J Chin Med.*, 2012, 40, 245-253.

[46] Lu, X; Siu, KC; Fu, SN; Hui-Chan, CW; Tsang, WW. Tai Chi practitioners have better postural control and selective attention in stepping down with and without a concurrent auditory response task. *Eur J Appl Physiol.*, 2013, 113, 1939-1945.

[47] Tousignant, M; Corriveau, H; Roy, PM; Desrosiers, J; Dubuc, N; Hebert, R. Efficacy of supervised Tai Chi exercises versus conventional physical therapy exercises in fall prevention for frail older adults: a randomized controlled trial. *Disability and Rehabilitation.*, 2013, 35, 1429-1435.

[48] Gillespie, LD; Robertson, MC; Gillespie, WJ; et al. Interventions for preventing falls in older people living in the community. *Cochrane Database Syst Rev.*, 2012, 9, CD007146.

[49] Zettergren, KK; Lubeski, JM; Viverito, JM. Effects of a yoga program on postural control, mobility, and gait speed in community-living older adults: a pilot study. *J Geriatr Phys Ther.*, 2011, 34, 88-94.

[50] Tiedemann, A; O'Rourke, S; Sesto, R; Sherrington, C. A 12-week Iyengar yoga program improved balance and mobility in older

community-dwelling people: a pilot randomized controlled trial. *J Gerontol A Biol Sci Med Sci.*, 2013, 68, 1068-1075.
[51] Patel, NK; Newstead, AH; Ferrer, RL. The effects of yoga on physical functioning and health related quality of life in older adults: a systematic review and meta-analysis. *J Altern Complement Med.*, 2012, 18, 902-917.
[52] Granacher, U; Muehlbauer, T; Bridenbaugh, SA; et al. Effects of a salsa dance training on balance and strength performance in older adults. *Gerontology.*, 2012, 58, 305-312.
[53] Krampe, J. Exploring the effects of dance-based therapy on balance and mobility in older adults. *Western Journal of Nursing Research.*, 2013, 35, 39-56.
[54] Jorgensen, MG; Laessoe, U; Hendriksen, C; Nielsen, OB; Aagaard, P. Efficacy of Nintendo Wii training on mechanical leg muscle function and postural balance in community-dwelling older adults: a randomized controlled trial. *J Gerontol A Biol Sci Med Sci.*, 2013, 68, 845-852.
[55] Munk, N; Zanjani, F. Relationship between massage therapy usage and health outcomes in older adults. *J Bodyw Mov Ther.*, 2011, 15, 177-185.
[56] Munk, N; Kruger, T; Zanjani, F. Massage therapy usage and reported health in older adults experiencing persistent pain. *J Altern Complement Med.*, 2011, 17, 609-616.
[57] Itoh, K; Itoh, S; Katsumi, Y; Kitakoji, H. A pilot study on using acupuncture and transcutaneous electrical nerve stimulation to treat chronic non-specific low back pain. *Complement Ther Clin Pract.*, 2009, 15, 22-25.
[58] Itoh, K; Hirota, S; Katsumi, Y; Ochi, H; Kitakoji, H. A pilot study on using acupuncture and transcutaneous electrical nerve stimulation (TENS) to treat knee osteoarthritis (OA). *Chin Med.*, 2008, 3, 2.
[59] Itoh, K; Hirota, S; Katsumi, Y; Ochi, H; Kitakoji, H. Trigger point acupuncture for treatment of knee osteoarthritis--a preliminary RCT for a pragmatic trial. *Acupunct Med.*, 2008, 26, 17-26.
[60] Yip, YB; Tam, AC. An experimental study on the effectiveness of massage with aromatic ginger and orange essential oil for moderate-to-severe knee pain among the elderly in Hong Kong. *Complement Ther Med.*, 2008, 16, 131-138.
[61] Hui, F; Boyle, E; Vayda, E; Glazier, RH. A randomized controlled trial of a multifaceted integrated complementary-alternative therapy for chronic herpes zoster-related pain. *Altern Med Rev.*, 2012, 17, 57-68.

[62] Palta, P; Page, G; Piferi, RL; et al. Evaluation of a mindfulness-based intervention program to decrease blood pressure in low-income African-American older adults. *Journal of Urban Health.*, 2012, 89, 308-316.

[63] Teut, M; Schnabel, K; Baur, R; et al. Effects and feasibility of an Integrative Medicine program for geriatric patients-a cluster-randomized pilot study. *Clin Interv Aging.*, 2013, 8, 953-961.

[64] Murray, MD; Morrow, DG; Weiner, M; et al. A conceptual framework to study medication adherence in older adults. *Am J Geriatr Pharmacother.*, 2004, 2, 36-43

[65] Krousel-Wood, MA; Muntner, P; Joyce, CJ; et al. Adverse effects of complementary and alternative medicine on antihypertensive medication adherence: findings from the cohort study of medication adherence among older adults. *J Am Geriatr Soc.*, 58, 54-61.

[66] Cherniack, EP. Complementary medicine use is not associated with non-adherence to conventional medication in the elderly: a retrospective study. *Complement Ther Clin Pract.*, 2011, 17, 206-208.

[67] Bell, RA; Grzywacz, JG; Quandt, SA; et al. Medical skepticism and complementary therapy use among older rural African-Americans and Whites. *J Health Care Poor Underserved.*, 2013, 24, 777-787.

[68] Maher, RL; Hanlon, J; Hajjar, ER; et al. Clinical consequences of polypharmacy in elderly. *Expert Opin Drug Saf*, 2014, 13 (1), 57–65.

In: Alternative Medicine ISBN: 978-1-63484-826-8
Editors: E. P. Cherniack and T. Holmes

Chapter 2

Alternative Worldviews and Health-Consumer Agency Are Associated with Use of Complementary Medicine (CAM) among Poorer Rural Consumers in Australia

Tass Holmes*
Anthropology, University of Melbourne, Parkville, Victoria, Australia

Abstract

Complementary and alternative medicine (CAM) is in widespread use among Australians. This chapter, diverging from demographic studies and professional naturopathic literature, presents the findings of an anthropological study in a small Victoria-state Australian rural community, designated 'Sephirah'. It explores CAM use by poorer residents of local townships, the provision of professional CAM to low-income rural people by practitioners, and the cultural and spiritual meanings and significance CAM held for research participants.

The study's findings suggest both self-prescribed and professionally-provided CAM are frequently resorted to by 'inner-rural' dwelling

* Dr, PhD

Australians, who often harbour alternative worldviews, linking CAM use for health maintenance to nature-oriented, non-mainstream political and spiritual beliefs.

Retaining a more-or-less marginal status relative to biomedicine, CAM nevertheless represents a health agency or activist position for many consumers who lack faith in the modernist biomedical approach, thereby contributing both to wellbeing and enhanced social-cultural identity. The sense of an 'inherent' CAM-linked agency is a refreshing discovery of the research.

Keywords: health-consumer agency, complementary and alternative medicine, folk medicine, women health providers, rural health and poverty

INTRODUCTION

'Non-medical' healthcare, usually termed Complementary and Alternative Medicine (CAM), is in widespread contemporary use across a broad spectrum of society, including in Australia (Morgan, Williamson et al. 2012; Maclennan, Myers and Taylor 2006). Contemporary surveys suggest a majority of Australians consume CAM regularly, representing a multi-billion dollar industry funded largely through out-of-pocket consumer payments (cf. Maclennan et al. 2006).

While demographic CAM research in Australia is largely concerned with understanding consumer characteristics (cf. Adams, Sibbritt et al. 2011, 2013), other authors engage with pressing issues of practice and professionalisation faced by practitioners (Bensoussan, Myers et al. 2004; Wardle, Adams and Lui 2010). The present chapter diverges somewhat from these literature trends, by describing some of the findings from an anthropological project focused on types of CAM selected by and provided to low-income contemporary rural-dwelling Australians.

Comprising participative fieldwork and semi-structured interviews in 'Sephirah', a composite Victoria-state small-town, the research documented extensive rural poverty in the study community, highlighting economic constraints to CAM access. For low-income consumers, a number of structural barriers were identified that limit access to private-sector healthcare. Similar restrictive effects impact the income-earning ability of CAM professionals, as private health providers.

Further to describing CAMs in popular use, and their economic context, the study noted consumer views about the cultural, political and spiritual significance of alternative healthcare, and explored a theoretical link between the choice to consume CAM, and its social and cultural locations. CAM use seemingly contributes to a sense of cultural identity, engendering a level of health agency or activism, that runs counter to its persistently marginal status in relation to biomedicine. Because a degree of health-consumer agency is often associated with the unconventional choice of CAM to support health, a polarised theoretical model was adopted to background the research, positioning CAM on one hand as marginal and on the other hand as agentic and activistic.

As outlined by several researchers (Goldner 2004; Bukovcan 2008; Flesch 2007), whose understandings were amalgamated into the theoretical framework of the research, an assertive position is commonly embraced by CAM consumers in conjunction with their adoption of alternative worldviews. Interviewee comments were found to reflect this sense of a CAM-linked health consumer agency.

Content of the Chapter

I commence this chapter's sections with a brief definition of CAM, an overview of the research methodology and theoretical framework, and a concise description of Sephirah's demographics. As a way of predicating the data, I then briefly review understandings about CAM from published literature (including CAM's relationship to biomedicine, consumer worldviews, and a positioning of CAM as encouraging health agency and activism), showing these sentiments are clearly reflected in the statements and experiences of research participants.

Two later substantial chapter sections follow. In the first, I summarise the overall research findings, under headings of 'commonly used', 'formalised' and 'informal' CAM types. I then present and explore major themes from the data that offer theoretical significance, recognising the coincidentally ancient and contemporary changing nature of CAM knowledge, the folk process entailed in alterations to popular health concepts, and a prevalent resistance against excess medicalisation and its limited appreciation of whole persons in domains of health, which may equate to an activist stance. CAM's alternativity is seen to offer considerable philosophical integrity for consumers deciding between healthcare options.

Defining and Situating CAM in Relation to Biomedicine, for Research among Poor Rural Consumers

CAM is a broad healthcare category, defined as 'complementary' or 'alternative' specifically in relation to biomedicine (Barrett, Marchand et al. 2003). It groups several modernised holistic non-biomedical therapeutic traditions (for instance, see Di Stefano 2006, who explains holism in naturopathy). For the research purposes, I defined CAM as *any* non-biomedical treatment, formal or informal, that aims to cure sickness, maintain or enhance wellbeing, or prevent illness. This permits inclusion of a highly diverse array of healing activities under the greater CAM umbrella.

Tovey, Broom and co-authors (2005, p. 3) state that, while 'traditional' medicine is characterised by its long history, cultural specificity, religiosity, and indigenous roots, CAM is better recognised by ideological or paradigmatic assumptions, of holism or naturalism, as well as by bearing a positional relationship to conventional biomedicine. Categorised as alternative (distinctly different or deviating from biomedical expectations) or complementary (an assumed helpful and useful adjunct to biomedicine), CAM purportedly remains inadequate to provide complete healthcare without 'primary' biomedical care, which is represented as always essential for health in modern western healthcare systems.

METHODOLOGY AND THEORETICAL FRAMEWORK

Design and Conduct of an Ethnographic Research Project

The research was essentially anthropological in nature, based on participative ethnographic fieldwork and interviews in the study community, a small town with a high proportion of low-income residents.

After ethics clearance from University of Melbourne HREC, fieldwork commenced June 2011. This provided a base-line indication of types of CAM in common use by local Sephirah people, and many useful examples of participants' alternative beliefs and politics, in the form of narratives, conversational content, and observed social behaviours, community events and lifestyle practices. Data from participative activities were grouped broadly according to types of CAM used, and component themes were drawn extensively from 54 in-depth semi-structured interviews. Interviewees were recruited by a purposive snowball sampling method – similar to that outlined by Broom (2009) in his study among cancer patients who use CAM – commencing with a known cohort of ‘intensive’ CAM consumers and practitioners. This recruitment method secured a group of highly passionate, articulate and involved respondents, who described several unusual methods of healing, and the cultural contexts, meanings, and value systems they associated with CAM, financial barriers they encountered, and the personal significance non-medical healing held for them.

The participant observation method was particularly enlightening, as social gatherings occasionally offered a stand-alone healing benefit. This was definitely the case for a poetry and song-writing group, which encouraged belonging, social support, identity, and creative expression.

With few exceptions, participants were each allocated pseudonyms. The possible limitation to small-town confidentiality was explained to interviewees prior to them signing a consent form. Interviews were digitally recorded, hand-written notes were made during interviews, and most were transcribed in full or large part by the researcher. Use of the town pseudonym ‘Sephirah’ for public contexts improves anonymity for participants who felt a need to speak freely without fear of exposure. Several naturopath interviewees, perhaps confronted with uncertainty through the experience of practising in a transitional or liminal zone of changing professional definition, midway between recognisably formalised and informal practices, insisted on their location being anonymous.

A Polarised Theoretical Premise

Throughout this research, I conceptualised and explained CAM-linked beliefs as potentially dichotomous or polarised, such that lived experiences associated with CAM use may occur in a situated way, at opposite, yet magnetically-attracted ends of a dynamic continuum. At one extreme, CAM users, including those with simplistic intentions of health maintenance, or an experience of improved wellbeing or cultural identification with specific healing methods, may experience an adverse emotional feeling or reaction through being labelled as ‘different’ or ‘deviant’, such as when alternative health choices are rejected and discouraged by a medical doctor, or due to social expectations of a normative biomedical approach to health. At the opposite extreme, embracing positive aspects of CAM consumption may constitute a significant part of an increased sense of health agency and possibly activism, that encompasses holism and rejects medical determinism.

CAM appears to offer consumers and practitioners a feeling of agency in health choices, of relevance for those with pre-existing or evolving alternative views. By virtue of the distinct paradigms and explanations for healing associated with CAM, its unique understandings about the 'psycho-physiology' of health, and its assumed ability to bring about healing or palliative relief when biomedical treatment is at times inadequate, the choice of CAM for healthcare offers a capacity to provide support for complex divergent spiritual notions and beliefs about human identity.

To emphasise the connection between diverse CAM healthcare choices and an alternative health agency or activism: One group of intensive CAM users openly discussed their non-mainstream ideas, tending to espouse an overt feminist stance that respects a sacred female or earthy creative spiritual energy, which they called 'Gaya', 'The Mother', 'The Goddess', or 'universal consciousness'. Their descriptions, such as, "I'm channelling the divine feminine Shakti energy", affirmed the power they perceived as inherent in this chosen philosophical position. Others claimed to be a witch, or said they practise 'white witchcraft', recognising this choice of an alternative identification alongside traditions of western herbal and energetic medicine, as a valid part of the territory of western occult spirituality. Some of these women made assertive or reactive claims that flew in the face of perceived negative labelling from conservative detractors, with statements like, "People think I am a witch, but they just don't understand anyway." These research participants associated agentic CAM-linked beliefs to spiritual concepts about human nature or identity, intertwining these further with understandings about women's rights, human rights, womanliness, motherhood, feminism, 'karma', construction of health through the expression of personal agency or 'power', and the use of unusual practices, including psychic healing, energy manipulation and Indigenous ritual healing.

This sense of CAM facilitating individual and group agency lent itself to the polarised but magnetic theoretical model, where labels of deviance and difference arising from the mainstream health policy field are applied to CAM, on one hand, while a positive activism and agentic approach to health, acknowledging CAM's long-established history and skills-base, its broad contemporary popularity, and clearly alternative politic, were equally apparent. The value of CAM as *different* or culturally unique finds connection with an intrinsic health agency, and reduced dependence on biomedicine, that comes of using CAM for salutogenic health maintenance. In this way, the initially imagined polar divide of this conceptual model resolved into a new conjunctive meeting point and starting position, encompassing diversity and alternative health-behaviours, and holding great value due to an embracing of CAM's cultural richness and traditional knowledge. For both consumers and practitioners, CAM now offers a 'new normal' in healthcare.

Explaining CAM's cultural locations by reference to a polarised and magnetic theoretical model of marginalisation and agency during this research facilitated a critique of the peripheral socio-political location of CAM in contrast to biomedicine, despite its widespread popularity and prevalence. It also enhanced an appreciation of the contributions of CAM to health agency, health activism and a salutogenic health literacy, running counter to the arguably more limited conceptual determinism that often characterises dominant medicine.

The Location and Research Participants

'Sephirah': Demographics of a 'Typical' Low-Income Rural Town in Victoria

Sephirah is one of a series of small towns strung along an Australian country highway, amounting to a population of several thousand, but offering scant employment opportunities for local residents. Sephirah postcode includes the sprawling remains of a historic gold and timber town, and a public housing cluster created through subdivision of an obsolete dairy farm. Many long-term residents of the area face entrenched poverty and hardship, with sole-parent households representing 26% of families with children (ABS 2013), and an estimated 40-60% of households depending on Centrelink welfare payments.

Warr (2005) has noted the familiarity of relational networks in poor marginal communities in Australia, and lack of opportunity for varied social experience and economic advancement. Poor living circumstances, common in rural towns (and urban public housing estates), are generally invisibilised in light of Australia's more usual portrayal as a first world country, whose citizens, often residents of large coastal cities and towns, live as middle-class consumers. 'Consumerism' is normative for much of the urban population, including in domains of wellbeing and healthcare provision. In contrast, people in rural communities, with higher rates of unemployment, are often unable to afford private-sector care including professional CAM, or private health insurance that would partially rebate consultation fees.

Australians living in poverty are defined as receiving a personal income approximating the 'poverty line' or less[1] (MIAESR 2013). Australia's poor are mainly welfare recipients, including sole parents (who comprise an estimated 16-30% of families with children, varying by location (see census data: ABS 2013)), and long-term unemployed, disabled, mentally ill, youth and students, many rural residents, migrants, Indigenous, and an expanding population of elderly pensioners. Long-term poverty is difficult to reverse in rural places, due to limited access to post-school education or employment.

Social and Economic Challenges of Life in Sephirah

In a cameo cluster of 70 households in a poorer part of Sephirah, near an ex-public housing estate, almost 56% of households received Centrelink welfare payments, and a high 26% were sole parent families (that is 26% of households documented, rather than 26% of families with children, mentioned above). Only a quarter included household members with post-secondary training, certificates, trades or university studies. Many non-welfare working class folk received minimal or low wages when employed, or had limited employment hours, and spent a sizeable portion of their earnings on costs of petrol, vehicle maintenance and expenses incurred travelling to urban employment.

In Sephirah, as in rural Australia as a whole, alongside welfare dependence there is widespread unemployment, moderate substance-abuse, an elevated number of suicides and homicides, and an over-frequent incidence of chronic disease and early deaths related to lifestyle problems (Dade Smith 2007; Lockie and Bourke 2001, pp. 105-108). Many rural people are chronically poor, effectively comprising part of an Australian 'welfare class'. Median family and household incomes in Sephirah are approximately $550 less per week than all Victorian and Australian households (ABS 2013). Low-income research participants described frequent transport problems, difficulty affording general living expenses, health issues, disabilities, and the experience of stigma attached to poverty.

By way of example, one 48-year old interviewee, Abelle, was married, with four school-aged children. Her income consisted of Centrelink partnered

[1] Australia's poverty line is defined as individual income of half or less of median employed income (median income is currently about $45,000/*per annum*, substantially less than average full-time earnings, over $72,000/pa). The poverty line, at half the median, is not much above $20,000/pa, and individual welfare incomes are less again.

parenting payment, and family allowance. With her growing family, Abelle lived in ten houses during the foregoing 15-year period. Although they had managed to buy a small steep property on a dirt road, they had neither spare time or money to build there, and were struggling to pay rates and afford costs of the children's education. When interviewed, Abelle was living in a \$275/week rental house, without a functioning car, at the top of a steep long hill in a rural township, distal to main roads and services. She explained that her husband was unable to do heavy work, earned little, and could lose his benefit if he worked more hours. Abelle held religious beliefs that partly defined her lifestyle choices. She grew garden vegetables, consumed herbal pills and vitamins, and infrequently visited a chiropractor or sought naturopathic advice.

This brief background provided a snapshot socio-demographic description of the not-atypical rural town community of Sephirah, in Victoria Australia, where this research was conducted.

Building Understandings about CAM Use from Literature and Research Data

Understanding CAM Consumer Worldviews

CAM's marginality (noted above) finds parallel with issues of rural health, and the status of rural populations, who have a greater acknowledged need for health services (Morrell, Kiem et al. 2014), yet are inconsistently funded by governments. This may contribute to a somewhat higher rate of CAM use among rural residents (Robinson and Chesters 2008; Adams et al. 2013). In general, published research about CAM consumers indicates they are mainly women, often with alternative or postmodern politics, a felt affinity with nature, and desire to participate in their own health maintenance (cf. Flesch 2007; Siahpush 1999; Lupton 1997). During the present study, some rural participant responses to questions about the character of CAM and biomedicine, as a rationale for their choice of CAM, illustrate a contention that CAM is perceived by consumers as distinct from biomedicine.

For instance, in stark contrast to normative formulations of health, one woman explained a preference for CAM, and her usual rejection of biomedicine, on the basis of popular 'lay' understandings that refer to the natural world. She said:

> I see western medicine as [like] what we do to the earth, you know ... [whereas CAM, such as] Chinese medicine, [depends on] working with nature; it's a whole philosophy, observing the body, seeing that [as a reflection of] nature ... work[ing] with ... the earth, not against it. [But] western medicine is like what *we* do. We screw with the earth, forcing our way in, changing things, thinking we know better. That's ... not listening, or it's arrogance, or 'we know better' ... And there's no connection.
>
> So ... they're just ripping out [body parts] 'cause they think that'll fix it, rather than seeing the body as a whole. ... I [believe western medicine/biomedicine] is very masculine, it doesn't have the masculine and feminine [balanced].

Such ideas, emerging from the research data, led me to a closer consideration of CAM consumer views and motivations, presented in the literature.

An Australian study of women with genetic predisposition to breast cancer (Field et al. 2009) found women who relied on CAM were active, educated, non-smokers and health conscious, but didn't attempt to use CAM preventatively because they felt 'at risk' and dependent on biomedical reassurance. This reflects common understandings of cancerous disease as a leading killer. Nevertheless, 12 percent of respondents in a Canadian study (Sirois 2008) consumed CAM without concurrent dependence on conventional medicine.

Robinson, Chesters and Cooper (2007, p. 113) suggest CAM is so popular as to be considered 'mainstream', with consumers valuing natural attributes of CAM, and having 'rurality' characteristics and an interest in spirituality, community, and exploring treatments that fall beyond the bounds of conventional medicine, to meet self-assessed health needs. Alternative worldviews appear a more significant 'pull factor' for CAM use (Sirois 2008; Siahpush 1999) than 'push factors' such as dissatisfaction with reductionism, doctor-patient interactions, or conventional treatment outcomes. Consumers enjoy longer consultation times and a more caring atmosphere with CAM practitioners, believing they 'treat them as a person' (Lupton 1997; Brown et al. 1999). Some research does outline discordant sentiments of patients toward biomedical information provision, or outcomes (Little et al. 2007).

A 40 year-old unmarried interviewee of this research, Layla, included both 'pull' and 'push' factors when explaining the reasons she preferred CAM, stating that her nature-focused worldview was especially influential. Layla has multiple diagnoses, of depression, mental illness and chronic fatigue, receives

Centrelink disability support pension (DSP), and lives in a small rural town with her elderly father. She likened her alternative ideas – believing animals and trees are sentient, and the world is a living place – to Aboriginal cosmologies, and claimed 'depression' is a psychically-located impact or sense of despair about global destruction of natural environment and habitats. Believing 'aural phenomena' (such as 'hearing voices') are part of normal human experience, Layla refused to take anti-psychotic medications. Instead she received psychological counselling and acupuncture, and self-treats extensively with herbs, nutrition supplements, walking outdoors, and creative pursuits.

According to sociologist Deborah Lupton (1997), this type of 'self-possessed consumer' personification resonates with late-modern constructions of body and self, being an entrepreneurial enterprise contiguous with self-conscious approaches to life, in contexts where expert knowledges, including medicine and science, are open to public challenge. For educated people, an over-thorough compliance with biomedicine may limit informed and independent consumer choice, and "deviates from … notions … about [the] importance of the autonomous self … govern[ing] personal behaviour via reason rather than emotion" (Lupton 1997, p. 374). Consequently, such consumers may refuse recommended medical treatments, and seek alternatives, through a desire to retain their independence or a feeling of control over health decisions.

Australian migrant communities also persevere in using folk-cultural medicine (O'Callaghan and Quine 2007; Dawson, Gifford and Amezquita 2000; Han 2000) that enhances identification with original culture. Retention of cultural or ethno-medical traditions may contribute to heightened criticisms of biomedicine (Bolton, Hammoud and Leung 2002; O'Callaghan and Quine 2007), and non-adherence to medical advice. Reassuringly, medical concern for the potential interactivity of CAM with drugs is not realised in terms of actual adverse effects of CAM being frequently reported (Welch 2001).

In Relation to Biomedicine: CAM as Activism and Agency

Theoretical appraisal of recent literature permits a view of CAM as nurturing of social activism and health agency (Bukovcan 2008; Goldner 2004; Long 2009; Pedersen and Baarts 2010), particularly for women (Flesch 2007). Naturopathy and CAM in general ideally recognise patients as thinking persons with unique problems. This orientation obligates individualised approaches (Di Stefano 2006) rather than routine diagnoses and treatments, and promotes health education (Long 2009), consumer empowerment, less dependence on costly or potentially toxic products of industry, and a reduced health-related 'footprint' (Hunter 2012; Litchy 2011). Engagement with CAM has come to signify a philosophical and practical resistance to biomedicine's pharmaceutical and pathology-oriented approach to managing illness, and mechanistic understandings of health and healing.

A comparison may be drawn, between counter-cultural activism generally and CAM's endurance, continuing to exist despite biomedicine's cultural dominance and the 'one-dimensional' perspective "that emerges in capitalism, that the system [in this example, the biomedical system] is a natural and inevitable phenomenon" (Ritzer 2000, p. 282). Promoting itself as necessary, and 'naturally' so, in any health context (Hodges 2011, p. 721), biomedicine seeks to displace the bulk of folk, traditional and indigenous ethnomedicine, engaging in ongoing processes of replacement, co-option or integration of 'other' medical knowledge. Hence, despite a trend of increased medicalisation of formal naturopathic practice (Evans 2008), CAM's perseverance as a diverse group of practices represents a field of agentic resistance and protest against the obliteration of traditional health cultures and healing knowledge.

Historically, Frankfurt theorist Herbert Marcuse believed the 1960s North American counter-culture movement and its activist protests offered hope for the future, because they bore witness to a broad and growing resistance against modern forms of social control (Farganis 2004, p. 397). Marcuse believed the alternative movement would ultimately save the world from destruction at the hands of capitalism and the 'juggernaut' of modern technology. Howard Becker (1973) later reconceptualised 'deviance' as a type of group defiance and a shared unwillingness to conform to unrealistic social expectations, thus giving rise to activism. Usually described through a 'conflict theory' lens, particularly Marxism, counter-cultural activism participates in generating 'social revolution' or 'class action'. Marx perceived revolutionary ideas, rather than being self-standing, were a product of the contextualising society, noting class struggles reflect and define society for a given period, and produce social change (Wallace and Wolf 2006, p. 85). These ideas established momentum for later social and political activist engagements.

Australian sociologist Raewyn Connell (2007) claims contemporary 'big picture' theorists, including Giddens, neglect genuine consideration of issues that hold importance for activists, feminists, and women consumers, and overlook the lasting impacts of colonisation on nations, Indigenous populations and minority cultures. Regrettably, while biomedical sprawl is described by some as a branching 'deep colonisation' (Hodges 2011; Bleakley, Brice and Bligh 2008), to date activism as part of western health culture is generally directed only toward improving access to biomedical or allied social support services.

Meanwhile, contemporary CAM-linked health behaviours arise from deep historic roots in the traditions of both western and non-western societies, and were markedly sidelined by biomedicine, in its role as a distinctively modern ethno-medicine, only during the twentieth century (Sherwood 2004; Jordan 1993). As such, CAM remains a 'natural' avenue through which a choice of holistic wellbeing serves to express dissent regarding biomedicine's underlying colonialist politics and its efforts to exert high-level control and surveillance over the lives of members of society (as theorised by Foucault). Against-the-grain theoretical (including feminist) positions construct activism as part of a representative 'voice' for social minorities, and may therefore fortify traditional health cultures, identities and knowledges. They hold relevance for understanding a CAM-linked health consumer agency, that enables better-informed and empowered consumer choices.

Naturopaths are recently described as enacting – through social engagement, advocacy, establishment of low-fee community clinics, disaster relief efforts and preventative and educational approaches to providing treatment – a high level of responsibility for human development and wellbeing (Tippens and Connelly 2007; Hunter 2012). Australian herbalist Assunta Hunter believes, particularly given lack of public funding support for CAM services, that this comprises an applied political activism, encompassing preventive education strategies that address social and economic determinants, of health and environmental concern, in addition to holistic nutrition and CAM treatment (2012, pp. 276-277). Few researchers have explored this idea in depth, of CAM as agentic, and effectively a part of the alternative-culture movement that runs counter to usual expectations of high-modern capitalist society.

The rural research in Sephirah incorporated information about values and meanings alongside description of the CAMs favoured by consumers and practitioners. Consequently, the data supplied numerous examples of CAM being used in a way that: (a) prioritises energetic, holistic and spiritual health beliefs in preference to two-dimensional, mechanistic or reductionist concepts, (b) places a high value on traditional knowledge, thus obviating a complete reliance on contemporary system-based 'diagnostic' health explanations, and (c) while *everyone* wanted more money, it also emphasised the importance that informal, locally-available and 'free' methods of healing held for poorer community members who valued CAM, in lieu of formal practitioner services, which remained unaffordable.

Grouped Themes from the Research Data

Three major themes were evident from the research data. I labelled these broadly as 'common uses of CAM', 'formalising CAM', and 'informal CAM'.

Common Uses of CAM

Despite most participants facing long-standing difficulties due to poverty, for example in sole parenting roles, they determinedly continued consuming various low-cost CAM treatments, and took part in healing activities to support their non-medical healthcare preferences, including yoga, meditation, healthful diet, community-based workshops, and groups such as 'mums support group', 'talking circle', or 'poetry reading'. CAM was used often for self-management of three highly medicalised conditions, being cancer, mental illness, and preparation for childbirth[2], all of which are usually overseen by medical specialists in oncology, psychiatry and obstetrics. Most consumers who self-prescribed CAM expressed agentic views about their right to self-treat, with remedies they felt were discouraged by medical doctors. Unsurprisingly, as 'inner rural' zones account for 22.5 percent of homebirths in Australia (AIHW 2010, p. 64), planned homebirths were common among Sephirah's CAM users.

Unfortunately, there appeared a discrepancy between a relatively good standard of wellbeing for mentally ill consumers who often used CAM, and a high number of local deaths of other mentally ill persons taking high-dose pharmaceutical medications (70 percent of a compiled list of known premature adult deaths). This may reflect greater interest in health-promoting practices among CAM users.

Due to unaffordability of private sector CAM practitioner services, some participants chose to access CAMs provided by 'integrative' GPs, who bulk bill, or whose fees permit Medicare rebates. Integrative treatments available included a limited few homeopathic or herbal medicines, and laser acupuncture. 61 year-old Helaina was not atypical among these consumers.

---

[2] These common uses of CAM will be described elsewhere, in forthcoming journal papers.

Helaina had used alternative medicine since she was young, inspired by becoming 'spiritually aware', and 'the metaphysics of health'. Long years of sole parenting and financial constraints had prevented her seeking professional naturopathic help for her children. Instead, she made dietary and lifestyle alterations, self-medicating extensively to improve her family's health, and 'purifying', "by eating very clean foods ... making ... yoghurt and living on ... fresh fruits and guava jelly." Recently Helaina was hospitalised after a psychotic breakdown. She settled in Sephirah some months later, and persevered with CAM to support her own and others' health, including conducting a talk circle for the benefit of local people. In an interview, Helaina recalled her two unattended homebirths (of four births), inspired by a 'spiritual calling', and many years of healing activities, including belly-dancing, herbs, nutrition supplements, special diets, massage, yoga, and chiropractic and acupuncture treatments. She now attends an integrative doctor for support and herbal extracts, and enjoys the rural location, for its "beauty and spiritual environment, all health-producing, [with] rainwater and fresh berries in season." For the flu, she had been taking garlic, lemon juice, ginger, echinacea, and olive leaf extract.

Contemporary co-option (Baer 2008; Singer and Fisher 2007) of isolated elements from CAM systems by 'integrative' biomedical doctors, such as 'medical acupuncture', or medical prescription of individual herbal medicines (the mild antidepressant western herb St John's Wort being the clearest example (Wahlberg 2008)), appears to increase the scope of medical practice (Possamai-Inesedy and Cochrane 2013). In Australia, this has led to a limited range of CAM being made available to low-income consumers through bulk-billing or Medicare-rebated integrative doctors.

Formalising CAM

A second theme centered on issues of professionalisation and formalisation of CAM practice, which is topical in CAM journals and published academic research. Consumers and practitioners of homeopathic medicine, naturopathy, Chinese medicine and community-based nutrition explained how they understood these healing systems to work, and practitioners detailed ways they seek to address health needs of poorer consumers.

Homeopathic understandings were centered on an energetic paradigm, of triggering healing by stimulating the 'vital force' using minute dosages.

Distinctions were made between the philosophy of homeopathy and other systems of medicine. Naturopaths focused on describing the nature of their practice, their provision for poorer clients, and ideas regarding possible regulation of practice. Chinese medicine practitioners noted an evolution in their approach, away from college-based learning and towards reincorporation of folk models that respect older philosophical understandings of body energies, and community-based practice structures that improve treatment accessibility. Consumers recalled experiences of Chinese medicine and how it improved their wellbeing. Nutrition practitioners were invested in community-level services, via a free food delivery, a vegetarian community café, and community gardens, all of which helped alleviate local poverty. In addition, a local allied-health clinic supported patients who were mainly referred by medical practitioners for dietary advice.

Informal CAM

A third theme, perhaps the most interesting from an anthropological point of view, concerned the common use of *informal* CAM practices. Anthropological literature discussing non-medical health concepts and healing methods arises mainly from non-western or non-first-world contexts, such as among Indigenous populations. Consequently, I was pleased to contribute to the literature by having observed and described a small number of contemporary Australian 'folk illnesses', and the way they were experienced and described by the group of rural-town residents. These include 'stuck energy', 'bad energy lingering around', having your vital energy 'drained' by another person, being 'unearthed', and experiences of 'burnout', 'sympathetic pain', or a 'coincidental' string of unfortunate events or illnesses.

Interviewees also elucidated some methods they popularly used to remedy these conditions, by 'smudging', ritual healing, psychic intervention, exorcisms and the like. In summary, informal CAM is in frequent use among residents of Sephirah community, and includes the following: (i) folk use of self-prescribed herbal medicine, both as a homely, crafty or wild/'bush-tucker'-related undertaking, *and* as a political, transgressive activity, that is loosely grouped by consumers with anti-capitalist or anti-consumerist views and applied in combination with a concept of 'witchcraft', involving psychic or ritual manipulation of energies to restitute healing and secure protection; (ii) the practice of psychic healing, white witchcraft, earth acupuncture (and less often, 'fortune telling', using astrology or tarot cards); (iii) alternative psychotherapy, mainly as 'narrative therapy', including Native American ritual approaches to healing; and (iv) hands-on and hands-off touch-based therapies, including various forms of massage, shiatsu, kinesiology, reflexology, energy channelling, energy balancing, laying-on hands and Reiki.

Several low-income participants frequently wildcrafted herbs from gardens, the bush or the 'nature strip', for health maintenance or to self-treat specific conditions, including hayfever, pneumonia, forgetfulness, insomnia, injury, 'toxicity', colds, flu, digestive problems, and localised infections. They each shared stories of being healed through self-prescribed herbal medicine.

One such consumer was Vida: In her mid-fifties, with a visual disability, Vida was an art-teacher for disabled adolescents and young adults. She lived many years on a part-DSP, and regularly commuted by bus, three hours each way for part-time work. In practical terms, Vida's main troubles were her low energy level, and transport problems. When feeling poorly, she self-prescribes flower essences, seeks counselling, deep breathes when walking outdoors, and includes herbs in all her meals.

Data from this research clearly suggests many CAM are in common use among low-income rural people, who cannot afford practitioner services. Furthermore, many diverse practitioners provide respected healing services that are poorly defined within recognisable professional boundaries of naturopathy, homeopathy, Chinese medicine and nutrition. Numerous less widely known therapies appear very popular among health consumers.

Unpacking the Significance of the Data

In seeking, through this research, to describe or characterise CAM by reference to participant beliefs and narratives, an important strand that drew together the themes that emerged throughout the data was a tangible link between CAM consumption and alternative worldviews, as the following passages highlight.

CAM is Both Contemporary and Ancient, and Incorporates New Understandings through a Folk Process

Practically speaking, contemporary consumers mainly use pre-prepared modern CAM 'products', in addition to conventional medicines. Some may be chronically ill and willing to try many treatments offering hope of a cure for challenging conditions. For instance, during this research, several participants with cancer diagnoses told of supporting their wellbeing over a self-treatment period that amounted to decades.

One interviewee, Bronagh, a petite divorced pensioner, recently died aged 73, after self-treating for a lifelong 'blood dyscrasia' cancer, that caused clots and tumours throughout her body. First diagnosed at age 19, Bronagh lived 54 years after doctors said she would die young. Like two other local long-term cancer survivors I spoke with, she subsisted on welfare payments for many years. Her use of CAM was predominantly by self-medicating, with herbal pills, extracts, diet, anti-oxidant liquids, and supplement powders or capsules. Bronagh accessed regular medical tests to measure chemical markers in her blood, and reluctantly took the prescribed drug Warfarin. However, she often refused other medical treatments, enthusiastically preferring herbal medicine. Bronagh brought an energetic outlook to community and family involvements, volunteering as a local radio announcer, and attributed her perseverance in older age to ongoing use of CAM, and refusal to comply with all prescribed or recommended medical treatments, which she believed were bad for health.

In contrast, adding a historical or archaeological perspective, recent research (Moore and McClean 2010) found traditional use of CAM as western folk-medicine is alive and well in the UK, including herbs, crystal healing, magical 'charms' and 'wool measuring'. Folk health beliefs and healing methods are retained mainly by people with simple lifestyles, in poorer rural and working-class communities, and by those who are frequently immersed in nature. Traditions of western healing are characteristically eclectic, incorporating beliefs and practices from diverse origins. These include treatments based on explanatory paradigms from European indigenous heritage, such as humoral (hot-cold) or nature-based cures (herbs, rest, breathing, respecting natural cycles, water- or sun-bathing), and spiritual healing, including prayer, faith or observances, psychic mediation, channelling of spirits and laying-on hands.

Another interviewee of this research, 41 year-old sole parent and Chinese massage student-practitioner Danielle, began bringing old-fashioned western esoteric concepts into her practice, having first absorbed these ideas into her personal worldview. She now amalgamates esoteric understandings with oriental massage techniques. Danielle spoke of her interpretation of 'the sacred feminine', describing non-physical aspects of her work with family members and massage clients as a form of energy channelling, situated within a greater sense of being and spirituality. She 'invites energy' into interactions with clients, suggesting this originates from 'spirit guides' and the natural world, and explained:

> [Healing, for me] is about finding my centre, and … working with the earth. … If I'm in tune with that rhythm I'm more centered. … It's kind of a 'paganistic' thing, connecting to that energy. … [Usually] I do a … prayer at the start, ask the guides to let me be a channel for love and healing, try and keep conscious of the crown of my head, be open to energies of earth and sky … and try not to get my head too involved. I visualise myself as a conduit for love and energy … to be open to it.

Such data, frequently encountered, evidence CAM's philosophical links to ancient historical bodies of healing knowledge or belief (cf. Brooke 1997), whilst also being used as supportive or adjunctive treatment in association with contemporary biomedicine. New understandings about healing, gleaned from individuals sharing ideas from their own learning, gradually become incorporated into a 'pan-CAM' belief system, through the effect of a recognisable folk process.

Reflecting this, popular beliefs about disease causation – such as emotional disturbances causing energy blockages that create sickness – were held by numerous participants. The concept of emotions causing 'blocked energy' derives, in contemporary parlance, from Chinese medicine theory. It provides a clear example of the lively folk process at work in the evolution of common understandings of health and illness, one that bears witness to changes taking place in the overall field of healing, of relevance to new knowledge and changed social circumstances. Two women who practised 'body-work' (respectively, shiatsu and 'EFT'[3]) each explained energy obstruction as a primary mechanism of disease pathogenesis, which was addressed and therefore cured by their preferred healing methods. Their descriptions highlight the ongoing incorporation of oriental beliefs into popular Australian perspectives about the way sickness begins, in this case as emotional and physical 'blockage', and how healing works, by resolving 'stuck' emotions that may trigger habitual kinesthetic and behavioural responses arising from a previous troubled time.

[3] 'EFT' is Emotional Freedom Technique, a brand of kinesiology treatment.

CAM Resists Widespread Excess Medicalisation, which Limits Appreciation of Whole Persons

Some research participants were deeply involved in living in a way they believed manifests an alternative philosophical stance, relying intensively on CAM as 'usual' healthcare. For those unable to afford CAM-practitioner treatments, this necessitated self-treatment and creative adaptation of simple cures. The value of preventive approaches, including self-care and community participation, was emphasised in the narratives of many low-income participants, who experienced benefits for overall wellbeing through involvement in community activities.

Lorelei, a grandmother with closely enmeshed local friendships and social networks, received oncology treatments for bowel cancer several years prior to her interview, and made a full recovery. Recalling her personal journey of healing, she highlighted the diversity of the many CAMs she had tried, and their suitability to her beliefs about astrology, the soul's path through life, and psychology. Lorelei mainly consumed homeopathy, western herbal medicine, Chinese medicine, raw juices and holistic psychotherapy, self-prescribed and through practitioner consultations, and eventually in conjunction with medical treatments. Her long hesitance in seeking conventional treatment reflected a fear that 'they' would "treat the symptoms only", thus disregarding her whole self and the meaningfulness she attributed to her experiential life journey. She believed a superficial symptomatic approach could suppress disease, potentially making it worse "at a soul level".

This belief, reiterated in various forms by other respondents, reflects that, from a holistic perspective, wellbeing or health is not about a singular fix for a specific diagnosis, but rather is an ongoing project, and part of a deep personal commitment to bettering both self and community throughout the entire life-path or journey. For many participants, undertaking long-term healing processes was viewed as essential for a meaningful life. These processes were experienced in steps or phases that signify changes in a whole state of being or personhood. In consequence of this idea – that wellbeing is part of a life journey – concepts of health and healing could not be neatly grouped into limited medicalised diagnostic categories, but were perceived as intrinsically multi-faceted and interwoven with other aspects of life.

I believe this finding would have remained less visible among a wealthier middle-class cohort of research participants. The low-income consumers, when desiring CAM treatments, were often forced to conceptualise, evaluate and prescribe for their own health problems, leading them to perceive health as one component part among their greater life challenges. Furthermore, this process of self-assessments and remediation takes place in challenging social contexts where their status and position are inherently political: Through being poor, they cannot help but realise the effect of structured inequities built into the capitalist consumer system, that impact on the quality of their lives and wellbeing (in terms of a cycle of poverty, an experience of stigma, discrimination and marginalisation, and a perception of the 'stress level' they face).

CAM Resonates with Alternative Views, and Is a Choice that Represents Integrity

CAM choice resonates with alternative philosophy or belief systems, and thereby may reinforce a counter-cultural outlook and sense of autonomous agency or political activism for health consumers. CAM consumers often espouse a way of life incorporating alternative worldviews and holistic health concepts, expressing the opinion that they have a right to freely choose healthcare suited to their own culture and beliefs. A choice of CAM therefore represents a feeling of integrity for many consumers, related to self-concept and social identity. This view appears especially prevalent among those *frequently* using CAM, as a core healthcare activity.

Integrity was important for 59 year-old Jennifer, with longstanding bipolar disorder, who was unable to afford visits to a naturopath in recent years. She regularly consumed self-prescribed herbs, vitamins, and flower essences, in conjunction with anti-psychotic medications. Jennifer previously had acupuncture and Chinese herb treatments, with private health cover, prior to her divorce, and values highly the idea that CAM methods are 'natural' or 'close to nature'. Beside the increased autonomy of self-selecting CAM, this perceived naturalness reinforces her sense of integrity, and is harmonious with her beliefs. Jennifer said she had "overheard a rational objection" to the usual healthcare system being enmeshed entirely with surgical and pharmacological beliefs and practices, thus neglecting social and holistic aspects of wellbeing. She believes administrative barriers prevented her from freely obtaining treatments of her own choosing. Her appraisal of health-system factors as negative was influenced largely by successes using CAM, across the course of some decades, which she claimed helped improve mood, sleep, immunity and chronic illness.

Critiqueing the healthcare system status quo, Jennifer felt a degree of superiority and jealousy exists among biomedical professionals, that keeps them distanced from CAM professionals. She exclaimed: “Doctors see these hippy tree-hugger-type [CAM] practitioners as beneath their dignity!” Instead, she imagined an ‘ideal’ health system, in which CAM practitioners could be considered equal to medical doctors.

Discussion

Despite cultural marginalisation in modern western societies, the attribution of a benign ‘folk’ character when self-selected by consumers, and its perceived alternativity (for example through conceptual associations with notions of ‘pure healing’, spirituality, or occultism), CAM can never be an apolitical or categorically neutral group of practices. The fact of CAM being kept segregated from and a lesser cousin in relation to institutions of biomedicine, in terms of formal policy recognition, supportive funding, and practice locations – all reducing its accessibility – effectively serves as a type of biomedical boundary-keeping. As a political device, this protects the established status of the medical profession from inroads by CAM professionals (see: Derkatch 2012), by economically preventing less-well-off consumers from access to CAM services, and devaluing CAM knowledge (Singer and Fisher 2007). Because poorer Australians cannot readily afford private-sector healthcare, including CAM practitioner consultations, without Medicare rebates, this results in restricted access to a range of health services that arguably contribute substantially to improved wellbeing, and may be considered essential to alleviate suffering for some unwell consumers.

Ongoing marginalisation of CAM for policy and funding contexts depends on normative first-world assumptions about how health and medicine should be understood or defined, and on an expected profit-making capitalist-system location of usual first-world healthcare consumption patterns. In particular, CAM’s persistently marginal status hinges on a widely-accepted exclusivity being accorded to medical doctors’ ideologically-premised right to define and practice what is construed as ‘necessary’ medicine (Baronov 2008).

The research described in this chapter emphasises popular uses of CAM, in a way that recognises the ongoing vitality of nonmedical healing practices, at grass-roots levels in an Australian rural community. Popular health beliefs continue to evolve through a folk process, incorporating new explanatory concepts and modes of expression, and accommodating changed social circumstances, such as the current widespread use of Chinese medicine by westerners. The research findings suggest many people do also strongly associate CAM with *modern* understandings about health and wellbeing, perceiving CAM choice as appropriate to support biomedical treatments, in addition to honouring the very deep roots CAM has within historic bodies of knowledge and ancient healing systems. Participants' statements reinforce connections between the popular adoption and oral transmission of philosophical elements from ancient western cultural traditions, and contemporary interpretations of cultural alternativity or counter-culture, and link these to a choice to consume non-biomedical therapies as an important part of usual healthcare.

For many contemporary Australian rural consumers interviewed during this research, CAM therefore represents not only a pathway to health and a heightened capacity to experience wellbeing, but a coincident cultural and political expression of resistance against the inappropriate shadow of increasing medicalisation that occludes various facets of personal and social life.

CONCLUSION

Data from anthropological research described here suggest self-prescribed and professionally-provided CAM are widely used by low-income 'inner-rural' Australian people, who may harbour alternative worldviews, and readily link CAM healthcare to nature-oriented, non-mainstream political or spiritual beliefs and opinions. As a diverse group of non-biomedical health practices, CAM in Australia retains a more-or-less marginal status relative to conventional medicine, receiving no government subsidies and scant policy recognition. Yet CAM use has come to represent an activist or agentic stance, contributing to socio-cultural identity in addition to wellbeing, for consumers who lack faith in modernist biomedical approaches to healthcare.

Telling poor CAM consumers' stories, this research addresses a literature gap, about the relationship of low-income status to CAM use, lack of equitable funding for access to CAM services, and the cultural meanings and roles personal politics, values, and spirituality play in a choice of CAM, particularly when it is difficult to afford. Further research is required to delineate CAM policy frameworks geared to addressing low-income consumers' reduced healthcare access, and to describe the importance of alternative spiritual and political beliefs, whether as an accompaniment to or inspiration for a choice of CAM to support wellbeing.

REFERENCES

ABS, Australian Bureau of Statistics. (2013). *2011 Census QuickStats: Australia – Data and Analysis*. Links for specific local areas: 'Families – weekly incomes', and 'Families – family composition'. Available online at: www.abs.gov.au/websitedbs/censushome.nsf/home/quickstats, accessed July 2015.

Adams, J., Sibbritt, D., Broom, A., Loxton, D., Wardle, J., et al. (2013). Complementary and Alternative Medicine Consultations in Urban and Nonurban Areas: A National Survey of 1427 Australian Women. *Journal of Manipulative and Physiological Therapeutics*, *36*, 12-19.

Adams, J., Sibbritt, D. and Lui, C. W. (2011). The urban-rural divide in complementary and alternative medicine use: a longitudinal study of 10,638 women. *BMC Complementary and Alternative Medicine*, *11*, 2.

AIHW, Australian Institute of Health and Welfare, in conjunction with University of New South Wales., Li, Z., Zeki, R., Hilder, L. and Sullivan, E. A. (2010). Australia's mothers and babies 2010. Perinatal Statistics Series No. 27, Cat. PER .57. Canberra: Australian Government.

Baer, H. (2008). The Emergence of Integrative Medicine in Australia: The growing Interest of Biomedicine and Nursing in Complementary Medicine in a Southern Developed Society. *Medical Anthropology Quarterly*, *22*, 52-66.

Baronov, D. (2008). Biomedicine: An ontological dissection. *Theoretical Medicine and Bioethics*, *29*, 235-254.

Barrett, B., Marchand, L., Scheder, J., Plane, M. B., Maberry, R., et al. (2003). Themes of Holism, Empowerment, Access, and Legitimacy Define Complementary, Alternative, and Integrative Medicine in Relation to Conventional Biomedicine. *Journal of Alternative and Complementary Medicine*, *9*, 937-947.

Becker, H. S. (1973/[1963]). *Outsiders: Studies in the Sociology of Deviance*. New York: Free Press of Glencoe/Collier-Macmillan.

Bensoussan, A., Myers, S. P., Wu, S. M. and OConnor, K. (2004). Naturopathic and Western herbal medicine practice in Australia – a workforce survey. *Complementary Therapies in Medicine*, *12*, 17-27.

Bleakley, A., Brice, J. and Bligh, J. (2008). Thinking the post-colonial in medical education. *Medical Education*, *42*, 266-270.

Bolton, P., Hammoud, S. and Leung, J. (2002). Issues in Quality Use of Medicines in two Non-English Speaking Background Communities. *Australian Journal of Primary Health*, *8*, 75-80.

Brooke, E. (1997). *Medicine Women: A Pictorial History of Women Healers*. Hants: Godsfield Press.

Broom, A. (2009). 'I'd forgotten about me in all of this' – Discourses of self-healing, positivity and vulnerability in cancer patients' experiences of complementary and alternative medicine. *Journal of Sociology*, *45*, 71-87.

Brown, B., Barnes, J., Clarke, M., Medwin, L., Hutchinson, A., et al. (1999). Relatives' lived experiences of complementary therapies in a critical care department – a phenomenological study. *Australian Critical Care*, *12*, 147-153.

Bukovcan, T. (2008). Advocacy and Activism in Complementary and Alternative Medicine Research: A Croatian Example. *Anthropology in Action: The Journal for Applied Anthropology in Policy and Practice*, *15*, 35-42.

Connell, R. (2007). Southern Theory: The global dynamics of knowledge in social science. Crows Nest: Allen and Unwin.

Dade Smith, J. (2007). Australia's Rural and Remote Health: A social justice perspective, 2nd edn. Croydon: Tertiary Press.

Dawson, M. T., Gifford, S. and Amezquita, R. (2000). "Donde hay doctor": folk and cosmopolitan medicine for sexual health among Chilean women living in Australia. *Culture, Health and Sexuality*, *2*, 51-68.

Derkatch, C. (2012). Demarcating Medicine's Boundaries: Constituting and Categorizing in the Journals of the American Medical Association. *Technological Communication Quarterly*, *21*, 210-229.

Di Stefano, V. (2006). *Holism and Complementary Medicine: Origins and Principles*. Crows Nest NSW: Allen and Unwin.

Evans S. 2008. Changing the knowledge base in Western herbal medicine. *Social Science and Medicine*, *67*, 2098-2106.

Farganis, J. (2004, [1993]). Readings in Social Theory, the classic tradition to post-modernism, 4th edn. New York: McGraw-Hill.

Field, K. M., Jenkins, M. A., Friedlander, M. L., McKinley, J. M., Price, M. A. et al. (2009). Predictors of the use of complementary and alternative medicine (CAM) by women at high risk for breast cancer. *European Journal of Cancer*, *45*, 551-560.

Flesch, H. (2007). Silent voices: Women, complementary medicine, and the co-optation of change. *Complementary Therapies in Clinical Practice*, *13*, 166-173.

Goldner, M. (2004). The dynamic interplay between Western medicine and the complementary and alternative medicine movement: how activists perceive a range of responses from physicians and hospitals. *Sociology of Health and Illness*, *26*, 710-736.

Han, G. S. (2000). Traditional Herbal Medicine in the Korean Community in Australia: A Strategy to Cope with Health Demands of Immigrant Life. *Health (London)*, *4*, 426-454.

Hodges, S. (2011). Second Opinion: The Global Menace. *Social History of Medicine*, *25*, 719-728.

Hunter, A. E. (2012). Commentary; Naturopathy, Holism, and Critical Medical Anthropology. *Medical Anthropology Quarterly*, *26*, 275-278.

Jordan, B (revised, by Davis-Floyd, R). (1993/[1978]). Birth in Four Cultures: A Crosscultural investigation of Childbirth in Yucatan, Holland, Sweden, and United States. Illinois: Waveland Press.

Litchy, A. P. (2011). Naturopathic Physicians: Holistic Primary Care and Integrative Medicine Specialists. *Journal of Dietary Supplements*, *8*, 369-377.

Little, M., Jordens, C. F. C., McGrath, C., Montgomery, K., Kerridge, I., et al. (2007). Pragmatic pluralism: Mutual tolerance of contested understandings between orthodox and alternative practitioners in autologous stem cell transplantation. *Social Science and Medicine*, *64*, 1512-1523.

Lockie, S. and Bourke, L. (2001). *Rurality Bites: The Social and Environmental Transformation of Rural Australia*. Annandale: Pluto Press Australia.

Long, A. F. (2009). The potential of complementary and alternative medicine in promoting well-being and critical health literacy: a prospective and observational study of shiatsu. *BMC Complementary and Alternative Medicine*, *9*, 19.

Lupton, D. (1997). Consumerism, Reflexivity and the Medical Encounter. *Social Science and Medicine*, *45*, 373-381.

Maclennan, A. H., Myers, S. P. and Taylor, A. W. (2006). The continuing use of complementary and alternative medicine in South Australia: costs and beliefs in 2004. *Medical Journal of Australia*, *184*, 27-31.

MIAESR, Melbourne Institute of Applied Economic and Social Research. (2013). Summaries: *Poverty Lines: Australia* (online ISSN: 1448-0530).

In Melbourne Institute, Labour Economics and Social Policy, University of Melbourne. Available online at: http://melbourneinstitute.com/miaesr/publications/indicators/poverty-lines-australia.html#y2013, last accessed 18 August 2014.

Moore, R. and McClean, S. (eds.) (2010). *Folk Healing and Health Care Practices in Britain and Ireland: Stethoscopes, Wands and Crystals*. New York and Oxford: Berghahn.

Morell, A. L., Kiem, S., Millsteed, M. A. and Pollice, A. (2014). Attraction, recruitment and distribution of health professionals in rural and remote Australia: early results of the Rural Health Professionals Program. *Human Resources for Health*, *12*, 15.

Morgan, T. K., Williamson, M., Pirotta, M., Stewart, K., Myers, S. P., et al. (2012). A national census of medicines use: a 24-hour snapshot of Australians aged 50 years and older. *Medical Journal of Australia*, *196*, 50-53.

O'Callaghan, C. and Quine, S. (2007). How Older Vietnamese Australian Women Manage their Medicines. *Journal of Cross-Cultural Gerontology* *22*, 405-419.

Pedersen, I. K. and Baarts, C. (2010). 'Fantastic hands' – But no evidence: The construction of expertise by users of CAM. *Social Science and Medicine*, *71*, 1-8.

Possamai-Inesedy, A. and Cochrane, S. (2013). The consequences of integrating complementary and alternative medicine: An analysis of impacts on practice. *Health Sociology Review*, *22*, 65-74.

Ritzer, G. (2000). Sociological Theory, 5th edn. New York: McGraw-Hill International.

Robinson, A. and Chesters, J. (2008). Rural Diversity in CAM Usage: The Relationship between Rural Diversity and the Use of Complementary and Alternative Medicine Modalities. *Rural Society*, *18*, 64-75.

Robinson, A., Chesters, J. and Cooper, S. (2007). People's Choice: Complementary and Alternative Medicine Modalities. *Complementary Health Practice Review*, *12*, 99-119.

Sherwood, P. T. (2004). Evolution of Natural Medicine and Biomedicine and their Future Roles in Health Care. PhD Thesis. St Albans: Victoria University.

Siahpush, M. (1999). Why do people favour alternative medicine? *Australian and New Zealand Journal of Public Health*, *23*, 266-271.

Singer, J. and Fisher, K. (2007). The impact of co-option on herbalism: A bifurcation in epistemology and practice. *Health Sociology Review*, *16*, 18-26.

Sirois, F. M. (2008). Motivations for consulting complementary and alternative medicine practitioners: A comparison of consumers from 1997-8 and 2005. *BMC Complementary and Alternative Medicine*, *8*, 16.

Tippens, K. and Connelly, E. (2007). 'Poverty and Human Development': The Social Responsibility of the Naturopathic Physician. *The Journal of Alternative and Complementary Medicine*, *13*, 783-785.

Tovey, P. A., Broom, A. F., Chatwin, J., Ahmad, S. and Hafeez, M. (2005). Use of traditional, complementary and allopathic medicines in Pakistan by cancer patients. *Rural and Remote Health*, *5*, 4, 447.

Wahlberg, A. (2008). Above and beyond superstition – western herbal medicine and the decriminalizing of placebo. *History of the Human Sciences*, 21, 77-101.

Wallace, R. A. and Wolf, A. (2006). *Contemporary Sociological Theory: Expanding the Classical Tradition, Sixth Edition*. Upper Saddle River, New Jersey: Pearson/Prentice Hall.

Wardle, J. L., Adams, J. and Lui, C. W. (2010). A qualitative study of naturopathy in rural practice: A focus upon naturopaths' experiences and perceptions of rural patients and demands for their services. *BMC Health Services Research*, *10*, 1-8.

Warr, D. J. (2005). Social networks in a 'discredited' neighbourhood. *Journal of Sociology*, *41*, 285-308.

Welch, S. A. (2001). The Use of Complementary Medicines by Inpatients at St Vincent's Hospital Sydney. *The Australian Journal of Hospital Pharmacy*, *31*, 111-113.

PART TWO: PRACTITIONERS

In: Alternative Medicine ISBN: 978-1-63484-826-8
Editors: E. P. Cherniack and T. Holmes © 2016 Nova Science Publishers, Inc.

Chapter 3

NATUROPATHIC DOCTOR OFFICES IN ONTARIO, CANADA: THE RELEVANCE OF VISIBLE LOCATIONS AND PATIENT PROXIMITY

Stephen P. Meyer[1] and Anita Kieswetter[2]

[1]Associate Professor,
School of Northern Development/Geography Division
Laurentian University, ON, Canada
[2]Naturopathic Doctor, Waterloo, ON, Canada

ABSTRACT

With the use of an Ontario-wide dataset of naturopathic doctor (ND) office locations and a survey from patients of five naturopaths in the communities of Waterloo and Greater Sudbury, it is determined that NDs (like chiropractors and dentists) are attracted to the vicinity of high visibility areas, although somewhat paradoxically, the majority of patients are not concerned with their ND's location. High visibility areas include those on, within or near main roads, high traffic land use and high population density neighborhoods. In aggregate, the patients consider quality of service and reputation to be much more important than distance to an ND's office. It is speculated that the value of a high visibility location to a naturopath may vary by the ND's length of time in business, the possibility of appealing to less affluent populations and likely agglomeration economies advantages (that is, the benefits of clustering within a given space).

1. INTRODUCTION

Health care recipients must overcome distance in varying degrees. Whether travelling to a family doctor or using naturopathic services, it is customarily assumed that some patients benefit from being more proximate than others. Rural citizens are frequently portrayed as most penalized in terms of health care accessibility in many jurisdictions [1-8], but spatial accessibility differs amongst urban residents as well [6, 7, 9]. The distance that people travel for medical treatments and/or counseling is largely a function of the geographic distribution of health care locations and how well the aggregated supply of medical services matches the demand over space. As with most small businesses in which clients pay for services largely 'out-of-pocket', complementary and alternative medicine (CAM) practitioners (such as chiropractors, massage therapist, acupuncturists, homeopaths and naturopaths) will have at least a general sense of where actual and potential clients are located as this may impact profitability. Part of the business strategy may include locating in visible locations, with comparatively high traffic flows and population densities. In accordance with planned holistic strategies, most naturopathic doctors (NDs) offer an extremely wide range of complementary and alternative medical approaches and augment and/or replace functions carried out by allopathic medical providers. Given this variety in service, NDs vie for patient pools shared not only by other NDs, but by all health care providers in some respects. As such, profitability will also be a function of a naturopath's effectiveness and professional standing. Yet, given breadth of service and importance of reputation, are naturopaths significantly affected by their location? Is there evidence to suggest that they seek to be in high traffic and visible locations to reach the widest market potential, or does a 'reputable approach' negate some of this need? Correspondingly, are patients of naturopathic doctors sensitive to spatial proximity?

The spatial patterns of health care providers and patient proximity are not new considerations. Yet, a disproportionate amount of medical geographic research is allopath-based. Research on the spatial characteristics of CAM has been comparatively under-developed, but contributions to the literature are occurring for specific jurisdictions [10, 11]. For example, Meyer [6, 7, 12-15] has published papers on the geographic properties of CAM and covers a range of issues for the specific case of Ontario and/or cities within the province. This chapter adds to this suite of research by, first, focusing on the geographic distribution of Ontario-based naturopaths in terms of spatial visibility (as measured by accessibility to main roads, high traffic land use and high population density neighborhoods); and, second via questionnaire results, contrasting patient characteristics with distance from ND offices in the communities of Waterloo and Greater Sudbury.

2. The Emerging CAM Literature

Most of the research on CAM utilizes questionnaire data to understand the characteristics of CAM patients and CAM providers. The general consensus is that CAM use is linked: to being female, middle-aged and Caucasian; to having higher levels of education and income; and with chronic non-life threatening illness [16, 17]. Other studies have associated CAM utilization with: conventional medical sector dissatisfaction [18], lack of allopathic access in rural areas [8, 19, 20], good health insurance coverage [21], a strong belief in holistic and natural remedies [20, 22, 23] and health-promoting behaviours [24]. Questionnaire data have also been derived from CAM practitioners to better understand the characteristics and/or 'healing philosophies' of: acupuncturists, herbalists and naturopaths in Australia [25], chiropractors in Chicago [26], chiropractors in Ontario [27], chiropractors caring for children in the United States, Canada and Europe [28], homeopaths in the western US [29] and CAM practitioners offering cancer therapies within the British National Health Service [30]. With the use of UK-based questionnaire data, Andrews and his colleagues published a number of perception-based studies including: how CAM operators cope with being a small business owner [31], why nurses leave the conventional medicine (CM) sector in favour of CAM [32], the attitudes of CAM therapist towards the British National Health Service [33] and the pathways to becoming a small CAM-based business [34]. The vast majority of these questionnaire-based studies do not stress spatial trends. However, there are a few examples in which survey information is evaluated with more emphasis on 'geography'; such as in assessing and contrasting CAM use: amongst rural (under-served) areas [8], amid rural and metropolitan locations [23] or between wider geographic regions [24].

Beyond the use of questionnaire/survey data, there is an emerging literature featuring empirical research that utilizes actual and/or aggregated locations of CAM operators to deliberately emphasize geographic trends and relationships. For instance, regression analyses were used to: establish the statistically significant relationship between the number of naturopaths per county in Arizona and Washington and proximity to naturopathic medical school and population density [35]; show that overall health professional shortage areas are related to chiropractic practice volume [36]; predict alternative medical use in the Netherlands by settlement characteristics, patient traits and perceptions towards CAM and CM [37]; and show association between place-specific criteria in Ontario (such as urbanization, diverse markets and closeness to other CAM operations) with various types of CAM office frequency (chiropractic, massage, holistic, acupuncture, naturopathic and homeopathic) [14]. There is also evidence that the spatial pattern of CAM behaves in a contagious and hierarchical manner with diffusion from larger urban areas [38]. It has been demonstrated that ND certification will spread in a contagious fashion, from licensed states to adjacent or proximal non-licensed states [39]. With a general nearest neighbor analysis and a nearest neighbor hierarchical clustering procedure, it has been shown that CAM operators are significantly clustered within four intermediate-sized cities and appear to be affected by agglomeration economies [12]. Evidence also suggests that CAM displays a more even pattern across the urban-rural continuum in Ontario in comparison to CM and, via local spatial autocorrelation testing, that certain CAM- and CM-specializing municipalities cluster in identifiable areas of the province and are associated with community well-being indicators and urban density measures [6].

Most akin to this chapter's focus, Meyer considered the spatial distributions of acupuncture, naturopath and chiropractor (combined) and dentist offices throughout metropolitan Toronto and categorized each point location based on visibility characteristics (as measured by proximity to main roads and commercial land use) and advertising tendencies (as estimated by advertising budgets and the size of yellow page ads) [15]. Many of the offices are located in high visibility/high volume areas and pursue more aggressive advertising approaches to, it is assumed, attract new patrons. Another group of offices are in high visibility areas, but eschew high advertising approaches; and on occasion the reverse is true (offices in low visibility areas, but with considerable advertising). There is a fourth group that locates in low visibility areas and has a modest approach to advertisement; perhaps, it is speculated, accruing revenues largely due to a strong reputation. In a general sense, the research described in this chapter builds on some of these themes by extending study on visibility to province-wide trends and more precisely assessing 'distance to ND office' tendencies with actual responses from patients. Along with continuing to explore distance and visibility issues in CAM, perhaps another notable rarity of this study is its use of both survey and actual location data within the methodology.

3. OBJECTIVES, METHODOLOGY AND DATA SOURCES

There are two main objectives to this study. First, geographic information system (GIS) and statistical analyses were performed to determine the extent to which 419 offices of NDs in Ontario are located in, or near, high traffic/high visibility areas. From the perspective of a naturopath's office, high visibility areas are assumed to be those that are most conspicuous in terms of traffic flow (vehicle or pedestrian) and are within, along or close to: land designated as commercial or governmental/institutional, high population density 'neighborhoods' and/or main roads. Commercial and governmental land use areas are planned for high traffic volume and therefore are more visible than other land use types (such as residential, industrial, parks and so on). In this study, high population density 'neighborhoods' are comprised of Ontario dissemination areas (small geographic units comprised of adjacent blocks) [40] that were in the top two quartiles of population density (or greater than 2,699.18 persons per kilometer for Ontario). Main roads include major highways, secondary highways and main streets [40]. For comparison purposes, the locations of 2,227 chiropractor and 4,684 dentist offices were also assessed in terms of visibility. These high visibility areas were identified within and outside of census metropolitan areas (CMA) and census agglomerations (CA) (see Figures 1 and 2) in Ontario. Queries to determine how many offices are within high visibility polygons, along main road lines or within 500 meters of these polygon or line features were carried out in the GIS environment. A Spearman correlation analysis was conducted to test the possible association between the percentages of high visibility ND, chiropractor and dentist offices located in Ontario CMAs/CAs. ArcGIS (version 10) was used for GIS functions and IBM SPSS (version 20) was utilized for statistical tests.

Based on surveys completed by patients of naturopaths, the second objective was to analyze if patient profiles differ with distance from an ND office. Two of these offices are located in the southern Ontario community of Waterloo (part of the Kitchener-Waterloo- Cambridge CMA) and three are in the northern Ontario CMA of Greater Sudbury. Patient traits such as reason for visit, mode of transport, age, gender and income were stratified by three spatial categories based on distance from each ND office. These categories are: 1) 'surrounding area' in which the patient is within the same or adjacent postal code polygon as the ND office, 2) 'outside surrounding area/within CMA' in which the patient resides in a postal code polygon that is beyond the surrounding area but within the same metropolitan area as the ND office and 3) 'outside the CMA' or that a patient's home address is in a postal code polygon located beyond the ND's metropolitan area. The survey results also provided supplementary information regarding the role distance may play in choosing a particular naturopath and/or health care provider. A digital layer of postal code polygons [41] was analyzed with ArcGIS to determine the postal code zone for the five NDs and their patients. A chi square analysis was performed to determine if patient attribute proportions, amongst the three spatial categories, differ significantly from an expected distribution.

The main dataset used for the Ontario-wide visibility analysis was purchased in August, 2012 from InfoCanada. It contains addresses, annual sales and other characteristics of naturopaths, chiropractors and dentist offices in Ontario. Telephone directories, annual reports and government records are the foundation of InfoCanada's databases, yet the company also telephone-verifies each case. It is possible, that up to 10% of the dataset may be inaccurate in some way [42]. The most common geographic error occurs when changes in office location take place between verification periods. The cartographic boundary files (dissemination areas, census metropolitan areas/census agglomerations, population centers, and provincial boundaries) [43] and road network files [44] were downloaded from the Statistics Canada website. The land use layer was obtained from DMTI Spatial Inc. [45]. The population density variable subsequently joined to the dissemination area polygon layer in ArcGIS, was obtained from Statistics Canada [41]. In ArcGIS, the address locator function was used to geocode the naturopath, chiropractor and dentist office addresses as points on to the road network layer. Points were agglomerated to various levels of geography (such to the CMA/CA or population center polygon layers) in ArcGIS. A CMA has a population of at least 100,000 with 50,000 or more residing in the core; while a CA has a core population of at least 10,000 [46]. A population center has a population of at least 1,000 and a population density of at least 400 persons per square kilometer [46]. These are 'urban' polygons and can be classified as: core, secondary core and fringe within a CMA or CA. Population center polygons can also be outside of CMAs/CAs. All remaining areas are 'rural' and can occur inside and outside CMAs/CAs [46].

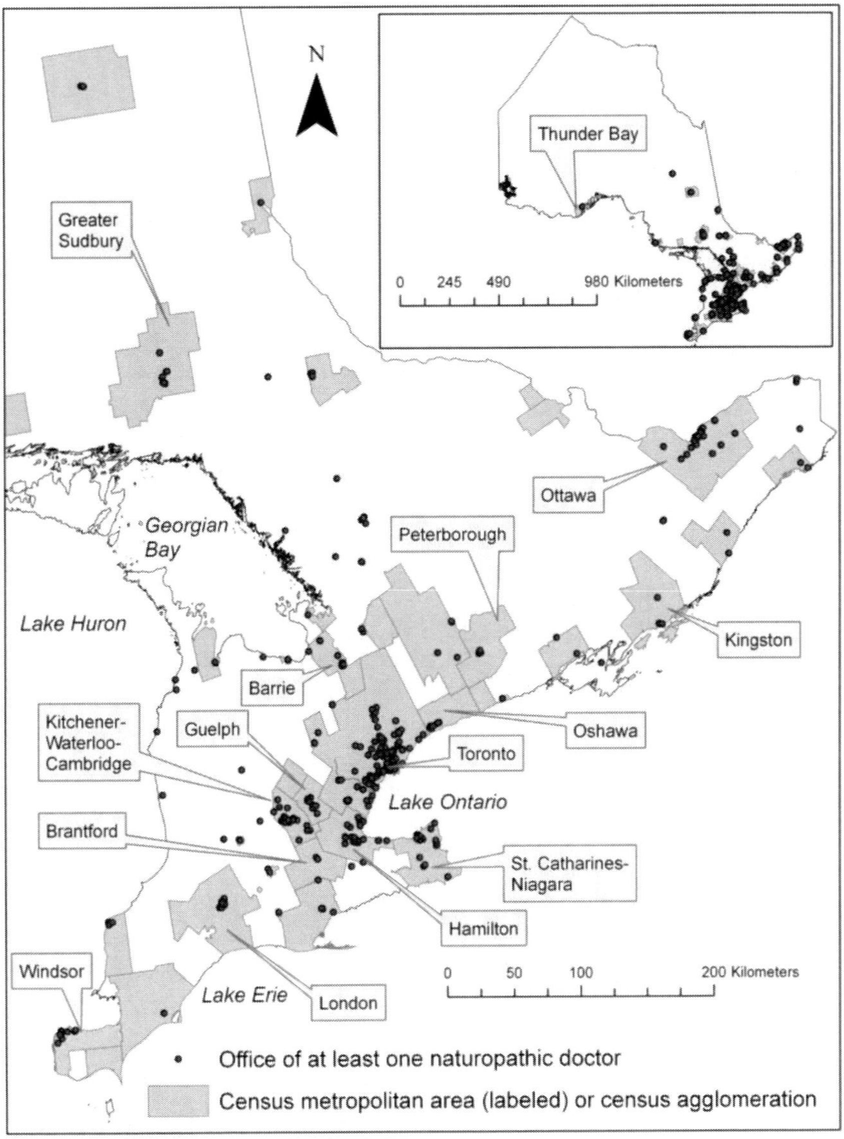

Figure 1. Census Metropolitan Areas (CMAs) and Offices of Naturopathic Doctors in Ontario.

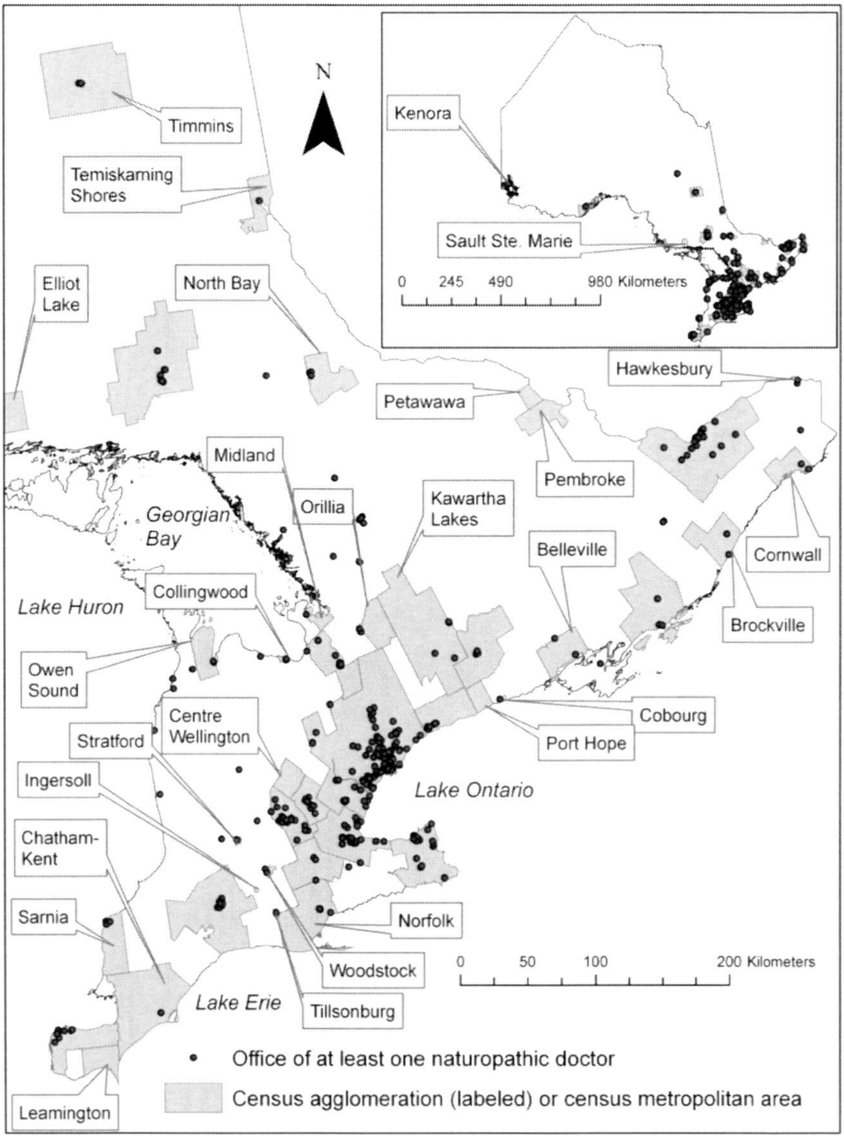

Figure 2. Census Agglomerations (CAs) and Offices of Naturopathic Doctors in Ontario.

The questionnaires for the Waterloo and Greater Sudbury portion of the investigation were administered through the offices of five naturopaths from

October 2012 to March 2013. In all, 96 questionnaires were completed and categorized with the use of ArcGIS and IBM SPSS. Patients were invited to check off basic biography information (age, gender and so on) and to elaborate on open-ended questions that gauged their opinions regarding distance/time travelled to naturopaths and/or health care providers. The surveys also contained questions on possible benefits and barriers for greater integration between health care providers; this information will be used to supplement a future study.

4. RESULTS

4.1. Offices of Naturopathic Doctors: Ontario-Wide Patterns and Visibility Trends

Figures 1 and 2 not only show the locations of CMAs and CAs in Ontario, but demonstrate the pattern of 419 ND offices throughout the province. While a few points are located outside of CMAs or CAs, an overall clustered geography is demonstrated with the most populated areas of the province (such as the Greater Toronto and Ottawa areas and more generally the south-central part of the province) housing a disproportionate amount of ND offices. Table 1 provides a summary of the location choices of ND offices throughout the urban hierarchy in Ontario and, for comparison purposes, chiropractors and dentist offices are also displayed. Generally speaking the patterns are quite similar amongst the three types of health care providers, but subtle differences are detectable. Most of these practitioners are located in core areas within CMA or CA areas; all post proportions of 80% or better with dentists most polarized at 87%. Dentist offices are most likely to be in the largest population centers (79.6%), but the majority of NDs and chiropractors are located in these largest of urban settings as well (69.9% and 68.9%, respectively). At the other end of the spectrum, it is worth mentioning that naturopath proportions are highest (7.2%) in rural areas compared to the other two office categories. The intermediate categories do not show strong deviations amongst the health care provider types. Thus, as with other small businesses connected with serving consumers, an unevenly high quantity of ND services will be where numbers of potential clients are greatest; or correspondingly, where visibility and typically spatial accessibility will be highest.

Table 1. Naturopath, Dentist and Chiropractor Offices Compared by Population Center Size and Type

	Naturopath number/%	Chiropracto r number/%	Dentist number/%
Population center by type			
Core inside CMA or CA	344/82.1	1,783/80.0	4,073/87.0
Fringe inside CMA or CA	16/3.8	92/4.1	128/2.7
Population center outside of CMA or CA	19/4.5	184/8.3	228/4.9
Secondary core inside CMA or CA	10/2.4	75/3.4	123/2.6
Non-population center (rural)	30/7.2	93/4.2	132/2.8
Population center by size			
Large population center (100,000 or more)	293/69.9	1,534/68.9	3,730/79.6
Medium population center (between 30,000 and 99,999)	47/11.2	230/10.3	341/7.3
Small population center (between 1,000 and 29,999)	49/11.7	370/16.6	481/10.3
Non-population center (rural)	30/7.2	93/4.2	132/2.8
Ontario	419/100%	2,227/100%	4,684/100%

Figures 3, 4 and 5 demonstrate the spatial patterns of visibility across Ontario from the specific perspective of ND offices in 35 CMAs or CAs. Eight CAs of Ontario's total 43 CMA/CAs do not have an ND office and are excluded from the percentage categories. For most CMAs/CAs, the majority of ND offices were not located on land zoned for commerce or government/institutional land use and this was true for all districts of the province (see Figure 3a). In fact, all but five communities had 25% or less of naturopaths located in these land use zones. Yet, most ND offices in the majority of communities were at least within 500 meters of commerce and government/institutional land use (Figure 3b). Hence, NDs appear to be attracted to the *vicinity* of these high visibility land use areas more so than being specifically within. The situation with main roads is different. As shown on Figure 4a, many CMAs/CAs are populated with NDs that locate specifically along a main road; the south-central district is perhaps most indicative of this trend, but the other regions of the province are broadly similar. Moreover, all CMAs/CAs in Ontario feature the majority of NDs on or within 500 meters of main road and often the proportion is over 75% (see Figure 4b). Main road proximity is clearly important to many naturopaths in Ontario. The propensity for NDs to position within a high population density dissemination area provides a very mixed pattern. Figure 5a shows that all legend categories are reasonably well represented throughout the province, making generalizations about the spatial distribution difficult. The pattern becomes clearer when considering Figure 5b; as a slight majority of communities are home to naturopaths that are at least within 500 meters of a high population density dissemination area.

Regarding the measures of visibility collectively, there are a few individual CMAs/CAs that stand out. Over three-quarters of the naturopaths in 17 CMAs/CAs (or half of all of the 35 with at least one ND office) are in, or within 500 meters of, all three visibility criteria (see highest categories of Figures 3b, 4b and 5b). These communities are: Thunder Bay, Sault Ste. Marie and North Bay in the northern district; Kitchener-Waterloo-Cambridge, Barrie, Toronto, Oshawa and Norfolk and in the south-central; Belleville, Hawkesbury, Peterborough and Kingston in the southeast; and Sarnia, Stratford, Owen Sound, Chatham-Kent and London in the southwest. The overall importance of visible location to naturopaths is apparent; particularly being *close* if not *within* these locales.

Do visibility proportions correspond between naturopaths and chiropractors and/or dentists? While only low to moderate Spearman correlations coefficients (albeit often statistically significant) occur between naturopaths and chiropractors and naturopaths and dentists (see Table 2), broad-spectrum trends unite these three health care types. It is uncommon for NDs, chiropractors and dentists to be within commercial or government/institutional land use (particularly naturopaths), whereas the proportions rise for positioning within high population density neighborhoods or along main roads. Very large majorities for all three health care types are shown for offices within the 500 meter buffers; again highlighting the importance of being proximate to, if not actually inside, high visibility locations.

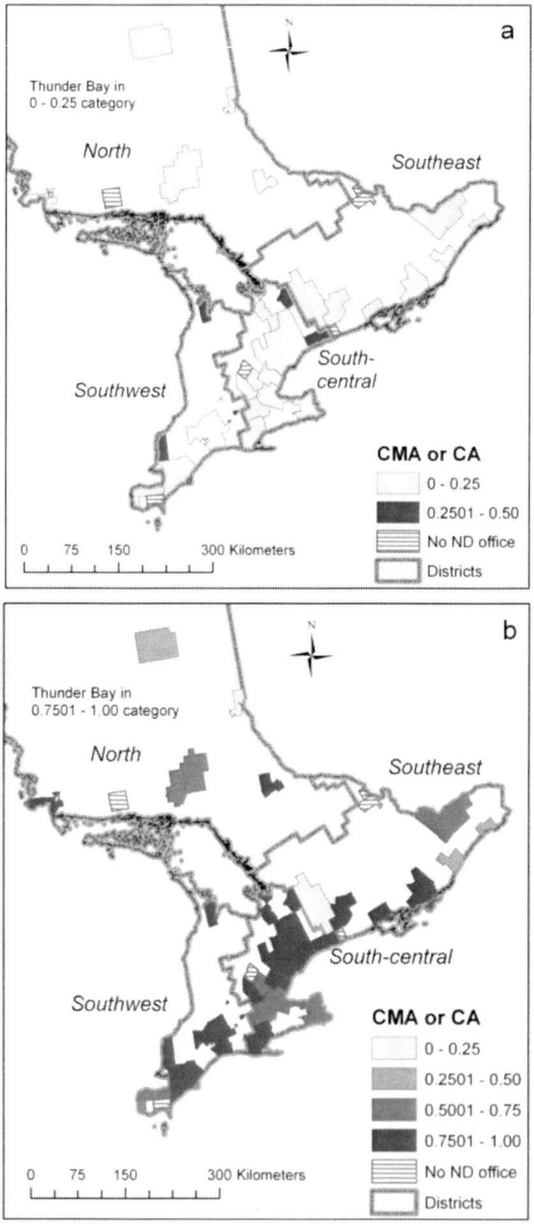

Figure 3. Percent of Naturopathic Doctor Offices in Commerce or Government/ Institutional Land Use (a) and Percent of Naturopathic Doctor Offices in Commerce or Government/Institutional Land Use or within 500 Meters of Commerce or Government/Institutional Land Use (b).

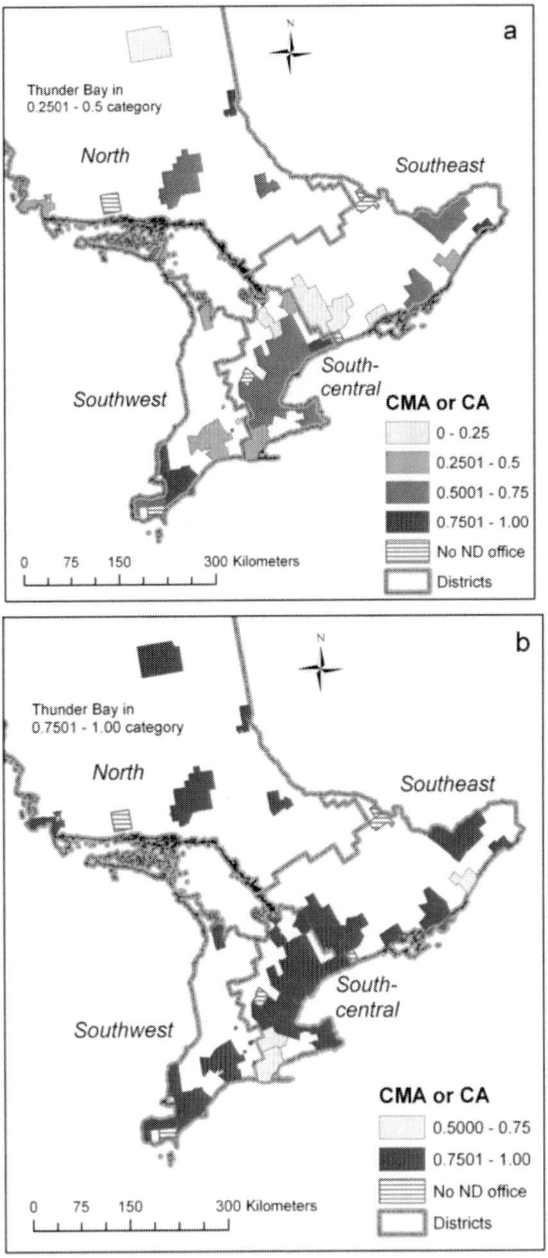

Figure 4. Percent of Naturopathic Doctor Offices on a Main Road (a) and Percent of Naturopathic Doctor Offices on a Main Road or within 500 Meters of a Main Road (b).

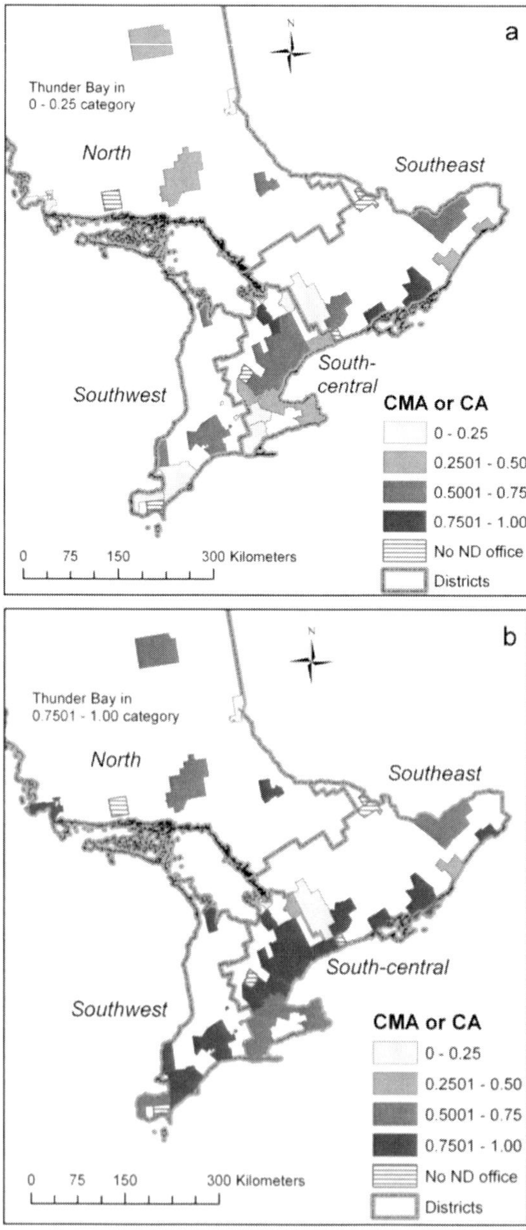

Figure 5. Percent of Naturopathic Doctor Offices in a High Population Density Dissemination Area (a) and Percent of Naturopathic Doctor Offices in a High Population Density Dissemination Area or within 500 Meters of a High Density Dissemination Area (b).

Table 2. Percentage and Spearman Correlation[1] Results for Naturopath, Chiropractor and Dentist Offices in Census Metropolitan Areas and Census Agglomerations

	All CMAs/CAs[2]: naturopath, chiropractor, dentist	Correlation naturopath/ chiropractor	Correlation naturopath/ dentist
Percentage of offices in commerce or government/ institutional land use	17.7, 22.0, 33.9	.41*	.24
Percentage of offices in or within 500 meters of commerce or government/ institutional land use	89.0, 82.3, 83.2	.51**	.35*
Percentage of offices on main streets	61.3, 67.3, 71.6	.37*	.51**
Percentage of offices on or within 500 meters of main streets	95.6, 97.2, 97.7	.36*	.25
Percentage of offices within high population density dissemination areas	56.9, 55.2, 64.2	.54**	.66**
Percentage of offices in or within 500 meters of high population density dissemination areas	84.1, 83.6, 90.4	.38*	.41*

[1] For the correlation analysis, N is 35 census metropolitan areas and census agglomerations with at least one naturopath, chiropractor and dentist office.

[2] CMA/CA percentages are based on 35 CMAs/CAs with at least one naturopath office and 43 CMA/CAs with at least one chiropractor and dentist office.

* Significant at 95%

** Significant at 99%

The subset of naturopathic offices situated beyond CMA or CA borders provides some distinctiveness, but visibility still has impact. There are 29 (of 419) ND offices that are located outside of CMAs/CAs in Ontario; 19 are within a population center (and thus still 'urban') and 10 are 'rural' outside of CMAs/CAs. Since these are chiefly more peripheral locations, it is not surprising that these offices are not associated with high population dissemination areas and are rarely proximate to commercial and governmental land use zones (although 7 of 29 are within 500 meters). Yet, it is common for these non-CMA/CA ND offices to be on a main road (14 of 29 or 48.3%) and virtually all of these offices are within 500 meter of a main road (26 of 29 or roughly 90%). Even in locations beyond metropolitan or built up urban areas, main road accessibility/visibly plays a role in ND office choice.

4.2. Naturopathic Patient Characteristics and Proximity Trends in Greater Sudbury and Waterloo

Table 3 shows age, gender and income classes across three spatial categories. Those visiting naturopaths were most likely to be in the 51 to 70 (41.7%) or 31 to 50 (36.5%) age groups. People outside of these 'middle aged' cohorts were comparative rare in terms of using ND services. Females make up the vast majority of patients; amassing over three-quarters overall. Regarding gross family income, sizable proportions of patients are in the higher income categories with \$40,000-\$80,000, \$81,000-\$120,000 and over \$120,000 categories receiving 31.9%, 25.3% and 26.4% of the total sample respectively. The family median income in Canada in 2010 was roughly \$55,000 [47] meaning that the majority of this sample would be above this 'benchmark'. It is also noteworthy that 93.8% of these ND patients travelled to their health care appointments by car and another 5.2% used a car at least some of the time. Given that ND services are paid for (in whole or in part) 'out of pocket', the common patient profile of being middle-aged and financially stable with car access appears to be logical. Table 3 also shows the results of chi square tests (for categories in which the expected value was high enough for reliability) and all were insignificant at a confidence interval of 95%.

Table 4 provides information regarding the reasons for consultation/ treatment and again there was no statistically significant link with the distance categories. The sample, taken in aggregate, does show that general health is the leading motivation for ND subscription (48.7%) with treating chronic conditions also making up a sizable proportion (roughly 30%). By comparison, it is rarer for patients to seek ND expertise for critical illness or for treating a new condition. That general health and chronic condition motivations stand out is perhaps not surprising given that the five NDs involved in this survey are, by-and-large, 'general family practices'. It is possible that in situations where a naturopath emphasizes specializations to a greater degree (women's health, oncology and so on), critical illness may be a more common reason for patient visits. Overall, this patient sample was quite evenly divided regarding single or multiple reasons for ND consultation. The notable exception is with those located closest to their naturopath in which case single reason visits were far more likely. One might speculate that spatial convenience may discourage a patient from 'accumulating' health issues before conferring with a naturopath.

Table 3. Naturopath Patients in Greater Sudbury and Waterloo by Age, Gender, Income and Location with Chi Square Results

	Surrounding area	**Outside surrounding area/within CMA**	**Outside CMA**	**Total (and %)**	**X^2 expected, X^2 statistic and significance (95%)**
Age					
18 - 30	4	7	1	12 (12.5)	4.0, -, -
31- 50	11	13	11	35 (36.5)	11.7, 0.2, No
51 - 70	14	16	10	40 (41.7)	13.3, 1.5, No
Over 70	1	3	5	9 (9.4)	3.0, -, -
				96 (100.0)	
Gender					
Female	21	30	22	73 (76.0)	24.3, 2.0, No
Male	9	9	5	23 (24.0)	7.7, 1.4, No
				96 (100.0)	
Income					
Less than $40,000	4	6	5	15 (16.5)	5.0, 0.4, No
$40,000 - $80,000	9	11	9	29 (31.9)	9.7, 0.3, No
$81,000- $120,000	9	8	6	23 (25.3)	7.7, 0.6, No
Over $120,000	8	10	6	24 (26.4)	8.0, 1.0, No
				91 (100.0)	

Table 4. Naturopath Patients in Greater Sudbury and Waterloo by Reasons for Visit and Location with Chi Square Results

	Surrounding area	Outside surrounding area/within CMA	Outside CMA	Total (and %)	X^2 expected, X^2 statistic and significance (95%)
General health	22	30	23	75 (48.7)	25.0, 1.5, No
Chronic condition	13	19	14	46 (29.9)	15.3, 1.4, No
New condition	8	12	4	24 (15.6)	8.0, 4.0, No
Critical illness	2	4	3	9 (5.8)	3.0, -, -
				154 (100.0)	
Single reason	19	19	13	51 (53.1)	17.0, 1.4, No
Multiple reasons	11	20	14	45 (46.9)	15.0, 2.8, No
				96 (100.0)	

The survey results also provided intriguing supplementary information regarding the possible link between travel distance/time and use of a specific ND. Of the 96 surveyed, 26 (27.2%) said ‘no’, without elaboration, to the inquiry: ‘Does travel distance/time influence your choice of health care provider? Why or why not?’ Another 50 (52.1%) of patients provided reasons for their ‘no’ response; these include the following.

1) I want ‘good’, ‘quality’ or the ‘best’ naturopathic/health care regardless of distance (29 responses).
2) I want to work with a ND/health care provider ‘I feel comfortable with’, ‘I have confidence in’ or ‘I trust’ regardless of distance (10 responses).
3) If the ND/health care provider gets results and helps improve my health, distance travelled is not relevant (6 responses).
4) Experience or reputation of the ND/ health care provider is more important than distance (5 responses).

The 20 patients surveyed that did consider distance as a factor are attracted to the convenience of proximate ND/health care providers (7) or are too busy to travel great distance (7). An additional six people of this group indicated that distance is only a consideration once a threshold had been reached (30 to 45 minutes). Thus, overall, the vast majority (79.3%) of the sample do not consider travel duration to their naturopath or health care provider to be consequential; particularly in contrast to other criteria such as quality of care and confidence in their ND.

CONCLUSION

This chapter provides evidence of an interesting paradox: collectively, naturopaths are sensitive to choosing, or being near, a site that is comparatively visible even though the majority of their patients would seek their expertise regardless of where they locate. Main roads, high traffic land use types (such as commercial and government land) and high population density neighborhoods attract a disproportionate amount of ND office activity throughout Ontario. That less multi-functional health care providers, such as chiropractors and dentists, show similar spatial biases in location preference is instructive. This suggests that NDs are representative of other health care practitioners, whose products and services are largely exempt from the publically-funded Ontario health insurance plan (OHIP), in terms of gravitating to the vicinity of high traffic/visible areas. Ironically, most of a naturopath's patrons seem unaffected by these high visibility spatial choices; as long as the service is good. ND patients in Greater Sudbury and Waterloo are most likely to: be female, middle-aged and comparatively affluent; seek ND services for relief from chronic conditions or to maintain good health in general; and drive to the ND office. This profile stays quite consistent regardless of where the patient resides in relation to the ND office. Moreover, patient consensus indicates that the reputation, effectiveness and demeanor of the naturopath appreciably outweigh any 'burden' one experiences from travel to treatment or counseling. So for the example of naturopaths, do highly visible locations only matter to the suppler and not the customer? This appears to be the case in aggregate, but some qualifying discussion is needed.

The priorities between an established naturopath and one who has recently entered the market may be quite different in terms of location choice. A new ND who has yet to establish a strong reputation and with a limited patient load may indeed benefit from being in highly visible locations to achieve 'walk ins' and generate name recognition from office signage. If this naturopath is viewed as an effective health care provider, with time their standing becomes enhanced and the need for a 'busy area' may decline. At this point, returning patients may be willing to follow the ND to other locations and new patients are gained predominantly through 'word of mouth' endorsements (and less so through visibility). With only five ND offices in this study, length of tenure versus location priorities could not be properly assessed, but this would make for interesting future study. The idea of therapeutic landscapes may have relevance. Therapeutic landscapes can refer to places that are conducive to healing, recovery from illness and maintenance of good health [48]. Although the notion of a therapeutic landscape is subjective, examples can range from formal spaces (hospitals, clinics and the like) to more informal places such as parks, churches and the home. It is common for naturopaths to fashion their office space in very tranquil terms often mimicking a typical home environment, but creating a 'healing milieu' outside of the office may be far more difficult in high traffic and/or dense areas. Perhaps this is why many NDs choose to be near, and not necessarily within, high visibility areas. Alternatively, a well established ND could certainly choose to locate in a more serene neighbourhood, perhaps at some distance from heavy traffic, and maximize therapeutic landscape benefits; whereas a new ND may forgo this option in favour of being highly visible.

Spatial proximity to health care in general can be particularly crucial for low income residents who, in additional to other challenges, may not have access to automobile transportation. Does this matter for the specific case of naturopathic care? As with other studies, the results herein confirm that ND patients tend to be comparatively affluent. This may partially explain why most people were not concerned about distance to NDs in Waterloo and Greater Sudbury; car access is almost universal amongst the respondents. Given that ND care is not part of OHIP and rarely completely covered under employee benefit packages, naturopathic appointments, procedures and prescribed products are paid chiefly 'out- of-pocket'. As a result, ND service may be unattainable for the least affluent; regardless of whether a naturopath is close by or easily accessible (on a main road with efficient public transit, for example). In Ontario, and likely elsewhere, a key challenge for naturopaths would be appreciably growing their client base beyond the middle to upper income classes. Certainly being spatially proximate to low income residents will help, but does this ultimately have significant impact? Policy-makers in many jurisdictions are concerned with spatial accessibility of all income groups to family doctors and other allopathic services. Should similar consideration be paid to CAM?

Another reason for the overall attraction of ND offices to highly visible locations may be due to the clustering tendencies of health care supply. Some naturopaths and other CAM practitioners gain from agglomeration economies (or the benefits of clustering in space). In some cases, naturopaths reduce overhead costs by sharing office space and staff with other CAM practitioners and possibly increase revenues as customer flow is enhanced with more health care professionals 'under one roof'. Health care clusters, comprised of diverse medical providers in close proximity, are likely to be in highly accessible and visible areas within cities. NDs, then, may be in high visibility locales not exclusively to grow patient loads, but also to be near other medical professionals. Is greater integration amongst CAM, and potentially allopathic, providers improved by spatial proximity? Health care clusters and the role that geography may play in fostering greater medical integration require further investigation.

Acknowledgments

The authors would like to thank Sarah Goulding, BSc, ND; John Bender, BSc, ND; Allan Price, BSc, ND; and Peter Jebreen, BSc, MA, ND for allowing the questionnaires to be filled out in their office space. We would also like to thank all of the personnel at Nickelridge, Pure Wellness and Health Coach for their help with the surveys.

References

[1] Arcury, T. A., Gesler, W. M., Preisser, J. S., Sherman, J., Spencer, J. and Perin, J. (2005). The effect of geography and spatial behavior on health care utilization among residents of a rural region. *Health Services Research*, *40*(1), 135-155.

[2] Rosenthal, M. B. Zaslavsky, A. and Newhouse, J. P. (2005). The geographic distribution of physicians revisited. *Health Services Research*, *40*(6), 1931-1952.

[3] Pong, R. W. and Pitblado, J. R. (2005). Geographic Distribution of Physicians in Canada: Beyond and Many and Where. Canadian Institute for Health Information, Ottawa.

[4] Langford, M. and Higgs, G. (2006). Measuring potential access to primary healthcare services: the influence of alternative spatial representations of population. *The Professional Geographer*, *58*(3), 294-306.

[5] Monnet, E., Collin-Naudet, E., Bresson-Hadni, S., Minello, A., Di Martino, V., Carel, D., Jooste, V., Cagnaire, A., Evrard, P., Obert-Clerc, B., Miguet, J. P. and Hillon, P. (2006). Place of residence and distance to medical care influence the diagnosis of hepatitis C: a population-based study. *Journal of Hepatology*, *44*(3), 499-506.

[6] Meyer, S. P. (2010). A geographic assessment of 'total' health care supply in Ontario: complementary and alternative medicine and conventional medicine. *The Canadian Geographer*, *54*(1), 104-122.

[7] Meyer, S. P. (2012). Comparing spatial accessibility to conventional medicine and complementary and alternative medicine in Ontario, Canada. *Health and Place*, *18*(2), 305-314.

[8] Hollenberg, D., Lytle, M., Walji, R. and Cooley, K. (2013). Addressing provider shortage in underserviced areas: The role of traditional, complementary and alternative medicine (TCAM) providers in Canadian rural healthcare. *European Journal of Integrative Medicine*, *5*(1), 15-26.

[9] Schuurman, N., Bérubé, M. and Crooks, V. A. (2010). Measuring potential spatial access to primary health care physicians using a modified gravity model. *The Canadian Geographer*, *54*(1), 29-45.

[10] Andrews, G. J., Wiles, J. and Miller, K. L. (2004). The geography of complementary medicine: perspectives and prospects. *Complementary Therapies in Nursing and Midwifery*, *10*(3), 175-185.

[11] Andrews, G. J. and Boon, H. (2005). CAM in Canada: Places, Practices, Research. *Complementary Therapies in Clinical Practice*, *11*(1), 21-27.

[12] Meyer, S. P. (2008). The spatial pattern of complementary and alternative medical offices across Ontario and within intermediate-sized metropolitan areas. *Urban Geography*, *29*(7), 662-682.

[13] Meyer, S. P. (2011). A spatial analysis of acupuncture practitioners in Ontario, Canada: assessing regional and intra-metropolitan trends. In: M. Saad (ed.), Acupuncture: Concepts and Physiology, InTech: Rijeka, Croatia, 189-206.

[14] Meyer, S. P. (2012). Place-specific explanations for the geographic patterns of complementary and alternative practitioners: contrasting chiropractic, massage, holistic, acupuncture, naturopathic and homeopathic operations in Ontario. *International Journal of Business and Social Science*, *3*(8), 24-39.

[15] Meyer, S. P. (2013). Evaluating the geography and the visibility tendencies of acupuncture treatment locations in metropolitan Toronto. In: L.L. Chen and T.O. Cheng (eds.) *Acupuncture in Modern Medicine, InTech*, 371-389.

[16] Bishop, F. L. and Lewith, G. T. (2008). Who uses CAM? A narrative review of demographic characteristics and health factors associated with CAM use. *Advance Access Publications*, *7*(1), 11-28.

[17] Manderson, L. and Canaway, R. (2013). Serious decisions: chronic conditions and choice of provider. *Qualitative Health Research*, *23*(12), 1638-1648.

[18] Avogo, W., Frimpong, J. A., Rivers, P. A. and Kim, S. S. (2008). The effects of health status on the utilization of complementary and alternative medicine. *Health Education Journal*, *67*(4), 258-275.

[19] Adams, J., Sibbritt, D., Broom, A., Loxton, D., Wardle, J., Pirotta, M. and Lui, C. W. (2013). Complementary and alternative medicine consultations in urban and nonurban areas: A national survey of 1427 Australian women. *Journal of Manipulative and Physiological Therapeutics*, *36*(1), 12-19.

[20] Meurk, C., Broom, A., Adams, J. and Sibbritt, D. (2013). Rurality, mobility, identity: Women's use of complementary and alternative medicine in Australia. *Health and Place*, *20*(1), 75-80.

[21] Steel, A., Adams, J., Sibbritt, D., Broom, A., Gallois, C. and Frawley, J. (2014). Determinants of women consulting with a complementary and alternative medicine practitioner for pregnancy-related health conditions. *Women and Health*, *54*, 127-144.

[22] Arcury, T. A., Preisser, J. S., Gesler, W. M. and Sherman, J. E. (2004). Complementary and alternative medicine use among rural residents in western North Carolina Complementary *Health Practice Review*, *9*(2), 93-102.

[23] Robinson, A., Chesters, J. and Cooper, S. (2007). People's choice: complementary and alternative medicine modalities. *Complementary Health Practice Review*, *12*(2), 99-119.

[24] Bormann, J. E. (2009). Predictors of complementary/alternative medicine use and intensity of use among men with HIV infection from two geographic areas in the United States. *Journal of the Association of Nurses in AIDS Care*, *20*(6), 468-480.

[25] Hale, A. (2003). 2002 Combined survey of ATMS and ANTA acupuncturists, herbalists and naturopaths. *Journal of Australian Traditional Medicine Society*, *9*(1), 9-15.

[26] Sarnat, R. L. and Winterstein, J. (2007). Clinical and cost outcomes of an integrative medicine IPA. *Journal of Manipulative and Physiological Therapeutics*, *27*(4), 336-347.

[27] Waalen, J. K. (2005). Practice patterns of 692 Ontario chiropractors (2000-2001). *Journal of Canadian Chiropractor Association*, *49*(1), 21-31.

[28] Alcantara, J., Ohm, J. and Kunz, D. (2010). The chiropractic care of children. *The Journal of Alternative and Complementary Medicine*, *16*(6), 621-626.

[29] Bell, I. R., Koithan, M., Gorman, M. M. and Baldwin, C. M. (2003). Homeopathic practitioner views of changes in patients undergoing constitutional treatment for chronic disease. *The Journal of Alternative and Complementary Medicine*, *9*(1), 39-50.

[30] Egan, B., Gage, H., Hood, J., Poole, K., McDowell, C., Maguire, G. and Storey, L. (2012). Availability of complementary and alternative medicine for people with cancer in the British National Health Service: Results of a national survey. Complementary *Therapies in Clinical Practice*, *18*(2), 75-80.

[31] Andrews, G. J., Peter, E. and Hammond, R. (2003). Receiving money for medicine: some tensions and resolutions for community-based private complementary therapists. *Health and Social Care in the Community*, *11*(2), 155-167.

[32] Andrews, G. J. (2003). Nurses who left the British NHS for private complementary medical practice: Why did they leave? Would they return? *Journal of Advanced Nursing*, *41*(4), 403-415.

[33] Andrews, G. J. (2004). Sharing the spirit of the policy agenda? Private complementary therapists' attitudes towards practicing in the British NHS. *Complementary Therapies in Nursing and Midwifery*, *10*(4), 217-228.

[34] Andrews, G. J. and Hammond, R. (2004). Small business complementary medicine: a profile of British therapists and their pathways to practice. *Primary Health Care Research and Development*, *5*(1), 40-51.

[35] Albert, D. P. and Butar, F. B. (2004). Distribution, concentration and health care implications of naturopathic physicians in the United States. *Complementary Health Practice Review*, *9*(2), 103-117.

[36] Smith, M. and Carber, L. (2002). Chiropractic health care in health professional shortage areas in the United States. *American Journal of Public Health*, *92*(12), 2001-2009.

[37] Verheij, R. A., de Bakker, D. H. and Groenewgen, P. P. (1999). Is there a geography of alternative medical treatment in The Netherlands? *Health and Place*, *5*(1), 83-97.

[38] Williams, A. M. (2000). The diffusion of alternative health care: a Canadian case study of chiropractic and naturopathic practices. *The Canadian Geographer*, *44*(2), 152-166.

[39] Albert, D. (2009). New York and Colorado as critical states in the diffusion of state licensing of naturopathic physicians. *Complementary Health Practice Review*, *14*(2), 59-69.

[40] Statistics Canada. (2012). Geosuite: 2011 Census. Statistics Canada Catalogue No. 92-150-XBB. http://www12.statcan.gc.ca/census-recensement/2011/geo/ref/geosuite-eng.cfm.

[41] DMTI Spatial Inc. (2012). CanMap Postal Code Suite. Markham, ON: DMTI Spatial Inc.

[42] InfoCanada. (2012). Canadian Business Directory: 2012 August Edition. Mississauga, ON: InfoCanada.

[43] Statistics Canada. (2011). Boundary Files, Reference Guide, First edition, 2011 Census. Statistics Canada Catalogue No. 92-160-G. http://www12.statcan.gc.ca/census-recensement/2011/geo/index-eng.cfm.

[44] Statistics Canada. (2011). Road Network File, 2011 Census. Statistics Canada Catalogue no. 92-500-X. http://www12.statcan.gc.ca/census-recensement/2011/geo/index-eng.cfm.

[45] DMTI Spatial Inc. (2012). Land Use (LUR). http://geo2.scholarsportal.info/.

[46] Statistics Canada. (2011c). Boundary Files, Reference Guide, First edition, 2011 Census. Statistics Canada Catalogue No. 92-160-G.

[47] Statistics Canada. (2013). 2011 National Household Survey, Geography Division, 2013. http://www12.statcan.gc.ca/nhs-enm/2011/as-sa/map-carte/thematic_download-hematiques_telecharger_R3-eng.cfm?SERIES=11&GEOCODE=1#DESC.

[48] Williams, A. (2002). Changing geographies of care: Employing the concept of therapeutic landscapes as a framework in examining home space. *Social Science and Medicine*, *55*(1), 141-154.

PART THREE: METHODS

In: Alternative Medicine ISBN: 978-1-63484-826-8
Editors: E. P. Cherniack and T. Holmes © 2016 Nova Science Publishers, Inc.

Chapter 4

A Brief Mindfulness-Based Meditation Intervention in Nursing Students: Report on a Mixed Methodology Feasibility Study

Jenny Jones[1,*], Mariyana Schoultz[1,†],
Angus J. M. Watson[1,2,‡] and Stephen J. Leslie[1,3,§]
Lecturer[*], Clinical Academic Fellow[†], Consultant Colorectal Surgeon[‡],
Professor, Consultant Cardiologist[§]
[1]School of Nursing, Midwifery and Health,
University of Stirling, Inverness, UK
[2]Department of Surgery, Raigmore Hospital, Inverness, UK
[3]Highland Heartbeat Centre, Cardiology Unit,
Raigmore Hospital, Inverness, UK

Overview

This chapter describes a feasibility study which assessed the effectiveness of a brief mindfulness stress reduction training programme in providing nursing students with a useful technique for improving situational (acute) stress-response resilience and reducing anxiety.

Abstract

Nursing students are exposed to stress when they undertake clinical placements and stress may be associated with increasing attrition rates in nursing undergraduate courses. Mindfulness meditation training has previously been shown to reduce stress in registered nurses. This chapter describes a mixed methods feasibility study which examined the usefulness and effectiveness of mindfulness meditation in improving situational stress-response resilience in nursing students. The chapter concludes by identifying recommendations for future mindfulness meditation research methodologies. Recommendations are also made for nursing undergraduate curriculum and undergraduate nursing student support services development.

Introduction

Nursing and allied healthcare professions are associated with higher levels of work-related stress caused by long working hours and the daily exposure to significant illness and emotional events [1, 2]. In addition, psychologists have hypothesised that a number of people who pursue healthcare careers may already have pre-existing higher baseline anxiety characteristics, resulting in greater reactivity to the stress-inducing challenges of the clinical environment [3, 4]. Analysis of workforce data on 30,000 NHS staff in 2008 showed that stress accounted for 15% of sickness absence compared to 4% in other public and private sector workforces [3]. In the healthcare worker population, stress is also associated with impaired professional performance and reduced levels of mental attention towards tasks, resulting in medication or other practice errors [1, 6].

Nursing students are particularly at risk of being exposed to healthcare work-related stress [7, 8]. Nursing students report higher levels of stress than senior medical students and the general population [9]. Up to 30% are thought to be experiencing stress levels severe enough to induce chronic anxiety and depression [10]. Stress may also be one of the factors associated with increasing nursing undergraduate attrition rates [11]. The unique stresses of nursing education have been found to affect both interpersonal effectiveness and academic performance [12, 13], regardless of personal character traits relevant to care delivery [14, 15]. As well as the new experience of exposure to traumatic illness events, the fear of making mistakes such as medication or treatment errors in clinical environments has been shown to affect concentration, memory tasks and problem solving abilities [7, 16, 17]. Over 30% of nursing students are thought to experience stress levels

> "…severe enough to induce mental health problems such as anxiety and depression" [10]

An inability to cope with clinical environmental stressors may not only adversely affect the student experience, but may also impact on the student's ability to deliver optimal patient care due to stress-related cognitive effects [18]. Which means an inability to cope with stress stimuli in nurse training may result in emotional disengagement, impacting on the student's ability to deliver safe and compassionate care during training and in future professional practice [19, 20].

'Stress' is often perceived of as a purely subjective emotional experience or described mainly in terms of psychological impact. In the Transactional Model of Stress and Coping psychological construct, stress is described as an environmental demand which has the potential to upset both psychological and physical wellbeing [21]. In this framework, stressful experiences are construed in terms of a relationship between a person's appraisal of a stressor and their available coping strategies used to mediate and regulate the stress demand. In contrast, the discipline of neuro-endocrinology describes the human stress response in terms of its physiological impact, the 'fight or flight' neuro-hormonal reaction [22]. Viewed from this perspective, prolonged stress demands lead to a long-term (chronic) adaptation of neuro-hormonal control mechanisms [23]. In this model, chronic stress has been associated with adverse maladaptation including altered cardiovascular regulation and distinct alterations in the hypothalamic-pituitary-adrenal axis production of the stress hormone cortisol. A growing body of neuroendocrine evidence suggests that there are associations between physical symptoms (including altered cortisol levels) arising from work-related stress and psychological symptoms of emotional exhaustion or a sense of depersonalization [24, 25, 26, 27]. This suggests that in some instances, those affected may not have adequate coping strategies to deal with the stress demands.

Given the work-related stress that nursing students are exposed to during their clinical experiences, the provision of training in stress management techniques and education is clearly needed in order to give optimal support to nursing students who are potentially vulnerable to situational stress and anxiety during their clinical placements [16]. As the nursing profession is such a high risk for emotional burnout and work-related stress, [1] preparing students by teaching them stress-reduction techniques at an early stage of their professional development may help the students cope more effectively with clinical work. And when employed, may also provide a potentially huge cost-saving benefit in terms of reducing sickness pay and bank staff costs to the NHS in the longer term. Therefore utilising one such existing validated and widely used stress-reduction program such as Jon Kabat-Zinn's mindfulness meditation stress reduction (MBSR) programme and testing its effectiveness and acceptability in nursing students may offer an adaptable and effective educational tool for students to use as a stress-reduction technique.

MBSR is a coping strategy that is said to encourage the practice of non-judgemental, moment-to-moment awareness in everyday life. The aim is to develop compassionate insight into one's cognitions or mental ruminations [16, 18]. Mindfulness meditation is said to be the cultivation of a state of mindfulness using specific meditation techniques. Its originator, Professor Jon Kabat-Zinn (2003) defines it as follows -

> "Mindfulness is the awareness that emerges through paying attention, on purpose, to the present moment, and non-judgementally to the unfolding of the experience moment by moment" [28].

Kabat-Zinn, a Professor of Medicine at University of Massachusetts Medical School, merged the concept of 'mindful' cognitive awareness and basic meditation and yoga techniques into an 8-week psycho-physiological educational programme known as Mindfulness-Based Stress Reduction (MBSR). This programme was originally developed for use in managing stress associated with chronic pain [29] but has been since found to be effective in a range of psychological and physical chronic conditions. These include the alleviation of depression and anxiety, reduction of pain in fibromyalgia and improvement in sleep-disorders [30]. The 8 week educational intervention has also been linked with an improvement in glycaemic control in type 2 diabetes mellitus [31], improvement of irritable bowel symptoms in women [32], alleviation of depression and clinical symptoms in chronic heart failure patients [33], more relaxed breathing patterns in women with heart disease [34] and a reduction in anxiety, emotional reactivity and decrease in the suppression of negative emotions in patients with heart disease [35]. Mindfulness meditation has also been shown to affect brain structure.

Anatomical Magnetic Resonance Images comparing an intervention group who had undergone the 8 week training showed increases in grey matter concentrations within the left hippocampus, posterior cingulate cortex, temporal-parietal junction and the cerebellum, compared to the study control subjects [36]. The MBSR programs offered at the Stress Reduction Clinic at the University of Massachusetts Medical School have now become the model for mindfulness-based interventional stress-reduction programmes at over 200 medical centres in the US and Europe [37].

This concept of mindfulness is not too dissimilar to the healthcare educational concept of reflective practice [30]. Reflective practice is meant to encourage the nursing or nursing student to develop a higher degree of self-awareness both 'within-the-moment' and 'in reflection.' The purpose of reflection is to become aware of habitual practices so that the practitioner can self-audit habitual thoughts, feelings and emotions for the purpose of improving practice [38]. NHS Scotland's "Flying Start" programme [39], designed to help newly qualified nurses progress through their first year of practice, offers the following definition of self-reflection –

> "…the gradual and continual process of noticing and exploring aspects of the self, whether behavioural, psychological or physical with the intention of developing personal and interpersonal understanding" [40].

So that reflective practice is

> "…embedded in our everyday practice in order to provide quality and holistic patient/client care" [34].

Therefore, given the integration of reflective practices as a core component of modern nursing education, there would appear to be a connection between Kata-Zinn's concept of being mindful in the moment, and the healthcare practice concept of 'self-aware reflecting-in-action.' This similarity suggests that mindfulness training may enhance reflective skills. More importantly, MBSR techniques may help nursing students develop stress resilient skills in the face of situational stressor [1]. This enhancement of stress resilience relies on the fact that the MBSR meditation technique involves the meditator learning how to maintain the conscious focus of their cognitive awareness so that they experience the immediate flow of events in their surroundings on a 'moment-by-moment' basis. The field of heightened awareness includes both external and internal events. The meditator focuses on their breathing pattern as a way of entering this heightened aware state. This increased heightened awareness on a moment-by-moment basis is said to allow the meditator to become conscious of subconscious ‘automatic’ or habitual thoughts, emotions and feelings. Once aware, the meditator adopts a form of cognitive dualism in their mind, becoming the watcher (or observer) of these habitual thoughts, feelings and emotions. When the meditator becomes consciously aware of these influences, they are said to be able to ‘slow down’ or calm the pace of their thoughts and by doing so, relax their psycho-physiological state.

This heightened awareness can involve noticing both mental and physical events. For example, someone trained in this technique may become conscious of an area of physical tension in their body (oftentimes an area of chronic physical tension) which they have not previously been consciously aware of [29].Mindfulness meditators differentiate the MBSR technique from other meditation techniques such as Transcendental Meditation precisely because they attempt to adopt a cognitive dualism, where the focused heightened ‘aware’ part of their conscious mind attempts to maintain a degree of separation or distance from the habitual thoughts and emotions that arise from the subconscious. Some mindfulness meditators liken it to watching a stream of thoughts pass by. These habitual thoughts, feelings and emotions are believed to be predominantly negative in content and therefore are seen as being the cause of acute and chronic psycho-physiological stress. Therefore mindfulness meditators aim to develop an attitude where they do not judge these habitual thoughts, feelings or emotions that arise, and instead, aim to cultivate a degree of self-compassion (from this dualist cognitive position), for any negative subconscious habitual thoughts or feelings that they become aware of [28].

The self-regulation of conscious awareness is thought to reduce psycho-physiological stress through the practice of cultivating a degree of cognitive distance from the habitual thoughts and feelings that the meditator eventually becomes aware of. The strategy is thought to lessen the psycho-physiological effects of these on-going habitual stressing forces. Eventually, the aim is that the participant applies the techniques to routine aspects of daily life in order to reduce psycho-physiological states of stress and anxiety [30]. Therefore key elements of the self-regulatory techniques appear highly adaptable to the acute situational stressors faced by nursing students in their clinical placements. For example, using a nursing student scenario where the student is administering drugs under mentor supervision to illustrate the mechanics of the MBSR construct, training in the MBSR technique should allow:

1. The student to recognise that they are stressed in a particular situation. For example, they may experience situational stress reading a badly written or confusing patient drug prescription sheet or when dealing with unfamiliar drugs. In such a situation, the student would become aware of physical tension, racing pulse, rapid breathing, negative thoughts about self-performance or capability etc.
2. The student would then be able to immediately respond by becoming consciously aware of their breathing (as trained to do so), slowing down their breathing and distancing their heightened cognitive awareness from the stressing thoughts, feelings or emotions that have been triggered in the situation
3. By becoming aware of their breathing rate and physical tension in the body on a 'moment by moment' basis, the student should then be able to recognise their habitual acute psycho-physiological stress response. And in doing so, view the psycho-physiological stress response without self-criticism (i.e., they don't get self-critical for becoming stressed, they just recognise that they are)
4. By recognising their habitual psycho-physiological response, the effects of this habitual response would be reduced. As a direct consequence, the immediate situational psycho-physiological response would lessen and their practice become more effective as a result of the self-reflection

Therefore the students could adopt the MBSR technique of moment-by-moment awareness when facing acute situational stress and link this self-reflection to reflective practice concepts. The MBSR skills could be instantly 'turned on' by the act of self-initiating a state of heightened awareness of breathing and cognitive focusing techniques in real-time, applied from the MBSR program. On this basis, we hypothesed that the MBSR techniques could prove to be a highly useful, relevant and appropriate stress-reduction tool for nursing students facing acute situational stressors in their clinical environments.

Previous research indicates that MBSR has indeed proved useful for nursing students, however the experimental measures of stress-reduction effectiveness have mostly been subjective and the MSR training courses have taken 8 weeks to complete. An 8 week mindfulness meditation intervention in Korean nursing students found a reduction in both anxiety (experimental group pre-test 44.93/post-test 39.38 vs. control group 38.69/43.74; p = 0.013) as measured by Speilberger's State Trait Anxiety Inventory, and stress

(23.69/17/27 vs. 19.5/21.4; $p = 0.020$), measured by the Psychosocial Wellbeing Index-Short form (PWI-SF) questionnaire [41] Baddoe et al. (2004) reported a non-significant trend ($p > .05$) of reduced anxiety as measured by the Derogatis stress Profile inventory following an 8 week MBSR program. Furthermore, as a result of participation, the majority of subjects reported that they returned to practice their MBSR breathing techniques at stressful moments [16].

As the majority of nursing students spend as much time in practical placements as they do attending university campuses for theoretical parts of their course, [7] a stress-reduction programme which addresses this unmet educational need would ideally need to be delivered in a form that is potentially more practical and useful for the nursing undergraduate curriculum. Which means it would have to be concise and adaptable to the shorter campus attendance schedules often found in nursing modular timetables. Mackenzie et al. (2006), using a novel 4 week version of the standard MBSR programme, reported a post-test subjectively reported increase in relaxation (experimental group pre-test 35.33; SD 8.95/post-test 43.56; SD 9.29 vs. control group 42.15 SD 9.94/41.00; SD 11.89; $p < .05$), Emotional exhaustion (26.38; SD 10.42/20.67; SD 10.39 vs. 16.15; SD 8.76/17.23; SD 10.62; $p < .05$) and job satisfaction (44.13; SD 8.38/47.40; SD 6.65 vs. 45.50; SD 8.98/45.92; SD 10.28; $p < .01$) amongst nurses and nursing auxiliaries as measured by the Smith Relaxation Dispositions Inventory, Malash Burnout Inventory and Intrinsic Job Satisfaction Scale [42]. These results suggest that a 4-week version of the programme may offer a more practical form of the training for undergraduate nursing students.

As existing MBSR research in nurses, nursing students and nursing auxiliaries primarily reports on subjective outcomes, experimental examination of the potential usefulness of a shorter form of MBSR training in nursing students would ideally include stress-related physiological outcomes. For example, to date, there has been no evaluation of the effects of MBSR on the 'fight or flight' cardiovascular stress response, which would help determine an objective measure of stress-reducing effectiveness. As MBSR makes claims to reduce stress, it is important to evaluate whether use of this technique can normalise the 'fight or flight' cardiovascular stress adaptation to help prevent chronic neuro-hormonal adaptation. A randomised controlled study evaluating a 4-week biofeedback stress-reduction training programme in police officers reported a significant pre-test heart rate increase in the control group ($p < 0.05$) in the face of a simulated stress test [43]. Therefore it appears that short-term cognitive re-focusing practices similar to MBSR can measurably reduce the 'fight or flight' stress response.

On this basis, we aimed to test the effectiveness of a shortened form of an established mindfulness meditation programme designed to reduce perceptual stress and anxiety states, based on the 4 week MBSR course delivered in the Mackenzie et al. (2006) study. We intentionally offered a shortened version of the trainng course in order to evaluate whether the reduced intervention length of 4 weeks (28 days) was as effective as the standard 8 week program in subjective outcomes. We also evaluated MBSRs effectiveness in reducing stress-related physiological responses. Therefore the study was unique in that it is the first to evaluate the effectiveness of a shortened 4-week (28 day) version of the standard 8 week MBSR programme in nursing students. It was also the first study to measure stress-related physiological outcomes as a means of assessing potential MBSR training-induced changes in stress-resilience to an acute event which aimed to emulate a transient clinical stressor experience.

Study Hypothesis

As Mindfulness Meditation is said to decrease anxiety and stress, we hypothesised that nursing students who receive a brief educational training programme in Mindfulness Meditation (4 weeks/28 days) (MBSR4) would show improved psycho-physiological acute stress responses and reduced anxiety levels compared to subjects in the control group. Also, given the difficulties nursing students face in campus attendance due to the unique structure of nursing undergraduate modular course design, we hypothesised that nursing students would be more likely to complete a brief MBSR training intervention programme. Therefore this mixed methodology feasibility study examined a brief (4-week) MBSR intervention (MBSR4) in nursing students using a validated psychological stress test tool in order to answer the following research questions; 1) Does completion of an MBSR4 reduce the transient cardiovascular stress response in the face of a psychological stress test? 2) What are the completion rates for an MBSR4 in nursing students? 3) Do participating nursing students believe that an MBSR4 is a useful stress reduction technique?

METHODS

Design

Randomised controlled single blind study embedded in a mixed methods feasibility evaluation.

Participants and Setting

26 nursing students (25 females and 1 male) were recruited from a School Of Health Science, University of Stirling, by an announcement to the whole class (n = 91). All participants were required to be aged over 18 years old, on no regular medication, had no previous formal meditation training and were able to give informed consent.

Intervention and Control

The intervention consisted of the MBSR4 (Table 1) [44, 45]. Intervention group members also received a CD of guided mindfulness exercises [46], session hand-outs and were asked to practice for at least 20-30 minutes daily (no measures of compliance were included in the study). Volunteers in the control group had no additional input other than usual nursing undergraduate course activities. There was a 28 day study extension to allow the control group the choice to also receive the 4 week training programme if requested.

Psychological Stress Test

Stroop's Colour Word Conflict Test (SCWT) was used to invoke a mild, temporary form of psychological stress, simulating transient psychological stress experiences in the clinical environment. Stroop's Colour Word Conflict Test is a widely validated psychological experimental stress test often used in laboratory stress research [47, 48]. It is designed to invoke a mild, temporary form of situational stress including a transient cardiovascular effect and the effects have been found to disappear quickly after the test has completed [49, 50].

Table 1. MBSR4

Program Component	Week 1	Week 2	Week 3	Week 4
Theme	Disengaging the automatic pilot	Dealing with barriers	Attachment and aversion	Developing and maintaining your own practice
Exercise	Mindful eating Body scan	Mindful stretching	Mindful sitting with awareness of thoughts	Body scan
Homework	Body scan Mindfulness of an everyday activity	Mindful stretching Mindful sitting with awareness of breath Paying attention to practice barriers	Three-minute breather Mindful sitting with awareness of thoughts Paying attention to likes and dislikes	Mindful sitting with awareness of breath and thoughts Continuing mindfulness practice

In this study, the test was meant to provide a simulated form of transient situational stress similar to the type of transient stress potentially experienced in the clinical environment, e.g., having to read a drug administration document under supervision of a mentor in a busy medical ward environment. To perform the test, the participant was asked to read out words representing names of some basic colours at a quick pace. The subjects were asked to read the name of the colour rather than stating what colour the words were printed in (e.g., the word blue was printed in green font). When reading quickly, people often become momentarily conflicted at the requirement to read the name of the colour rather than identify the actual colour the word is printed in, because cognitive learned inference influence their perception of the printed word [1]. The stress test was delivered at baseline, then 4 weeks later.

Outcome Measures

Heart rate (HR) and blood pressure (BP) were measured to evaluate the cardiovascular effects of the stress test. Transient self-reported anxiety was measured using Speilberger's psychometric State Anxiety Inventory (SAI) [51]. Mindfulness Attention Awareness Scale (MAAS) was used to evaluate the degree to which the participants maintain a heightened sense of awareness [52]. These psychometric changes were also measured at baseline, and then again at 4 weeks.

The feasibility and value of MBSR4 was evaluated by rates of attrition from participation in each week of the programme in the intervention and 'wait list' control groups. Also, through the use of a visual analogue scale (VAS) for intervention group participants to numerically rate the perceived benefits of MBSR4. The scale ranged from '0' - indicating that "*the practice was of no use*" to '10' indicating that "*the practice was very useful.*" The VAS is a well-validated method for measuring situational responses [53, 54] and we used centimetres (cm) for the measurement scale. Optional responses as free text and categorical data were anonymously collected at the end of the study using a free online survey invitation (surveymonkey.com) sent via student email.

The acceptability of the MBSR4 was evaluated by a study-exit survey. At the end of the study, all students in the intervention group were sent an optional link to an anonymous online survey (surveymonkey.com).

Sample Size

Little is currently known about the magnitude of any specific cardiovascular effects of MBSR4 or its transient impact on BP or HR in the face of a psychological stress test, therefore we used a pragmatic convenience sample of 26 volunteers.

Location

University of Stirling School of Health Sciences, Highland Campus, Centre for Health Science, Inverness, Scotland.

Randomisation and Blinding

Equal group random allocation was performed by a third party not involved with the study, using computer generated random numbers. Subjects were randomly allocated to either received MBSR4 or to the control ('wait list') group. Data analysts did not have access to the allocation list until data analysis was complete.

Procedure

Participants underwent the same assessment at baseline and at 4 weeks. All participants had resting HR and systolic (SBP) and diastolic blood pressure (DBP) measured prior to exposure to the psychological stress test (JJ), using a validated automated sphygmomanometer device (Microlife BP A200 Plus, Microlife, Germany) [55]. Two individual measurements were taken at 5 minute intervals to ensure less than 10% variation in measurements at rest and were then exposed to the psychological stress test for 10 minutes. HR, SBP and DBP were measured immediately after the stress test. Overall mean and standard deviation (SD) were then calculated for each set of measurements. All cardiovascular measurements and psychological stress tests were conducted in a quiet, draught-free room maintained at a constant temperature of 22–24^{0}C. Participants completed a SAI and MAAS questionnaire before and after the stress test.

Ethics

The study was undertaken with the approval of the Research and Ethics Committee, University of Stirling, in accordance with the Declaration of Helsinki. Written informed consent was obtained from each student before entry into the study.

Statistical Analysis

Paired 't' test were used to compare pre and post-test SAI and MAAS scores (Microsoft Excel Version 10, Microsoft, Redmond, Washington, USA and Minitab version 16.1.1.1. Microsoft, Redmond, Washington, USA). Data are expressed as mean and SD unless otherwise specified. Statistical significance was taken at the 5% level.

Results

26 students (mean age 31.7 ± 8.1 years) were recruited between July and August 2012, 9 (8 females and 1 male) and 35% (9) withdrew from the study, so were excluded from further analyses. Demographics and resting HR and BP measurements are shown in Table 2.

Table 2. Resting cardiovascular parameters at baseline and 4 weeks

	Control	MBSR4	p value*
Demographics			
Age	28.9 (6.3)	33.6 (9.4)	n/a
Gender	9 (female)	8 (female)	
Resting HR and BP			
Baseline			
HR (bpm)	80.5 (9.6)	76.1 (9.7)	0.06
SBP (mmHg)	116.4 (9.2)	117.2 (9.8)	0.40
DBP (mmHg)	75.2 (7.8)	75.2 (9.5)	0.49
4 weeks			
HR (bpm)	72.4 (9.2)	73.0 (14.4)	0.49
SBP (mmHg)	116.4 (8.6)	121.9 (14.9)	0.27
DBP (mmHg)	73.6 (8.7)	73.6 (10.8)	0.32

Mean (SD).

* paired t-test. Heart rate (HR), systolic blood pressure (SBP), diastolic blood pressure (DBP), beat per min (bpm).

Cardiovascular Outcomes

There was no change in HR or BP immediately after the stress test compared with rest (at either baseline or 4 weeks). Furthermore, there appeared to be no effect of the MBSR4 on resting HR and BP at 4 weeks (Table 3).

State Anxiety and Mindful Awareness Outcomes

There was no significant baseline vs. 4 week difference in perceived state of anxiety (SAI) scores (MBSR441.1 (9.0) vs. 38.3 (0.3), $p > 0.05$; Control 45.8 (14.3) vs. 42.5 (14.9), $p > 0.05$) or mindfulness awareness (MAAS

Scores) (MBSR4 51.0 (9.3) vs. 4 week 55.7(7.3), $p > 0.05$; Control group 51.0(12.1) vs. 54.1(18.6),$p > 0.05$).

Table 3. Effect of Stroop's coloured word test on heart rate and blood pressure. Mean (SD).*paired t-test. Heart rate (HR), systolic blood pressure (SBP), diastolic blood pressure (DBP), beat per min (bpm)

	Baseline			4 weeks		
	rest	post stress	p	rest	post stress	p
Control						
Heart rate	80.5 (9.6)	75.8 (11.2)	0.093	72.4 (9.2)	70.6 (9.6)	0.144
Systolic BP	116.4 (9.2)	113.2 (9.6)	0.351	116.4 (8.6)	117.0 (13.0)	0.793
Diastolic BP	75.2 (7.7)	72.6 (7.1)	0.314	73.6 (8.7)	71.6 (10.3)	0.261
MBSR						
Heart rate	76.1 (9.7)	75.4 (10.3)	0.554	73.0 (14.4)	73.7 (14.1)	0.518
Systolic BP	117.2 (9.8)	115.7 (11.3)	0.455	121.9 (14.9)	118.3 (12.9)	0.304
Diastolic BP	75.2 (9.5)	72.6 (10.6)	0.370	73.6 (10.8)	71.6 (7.3)	0.145

Feasibility of Using a Brief MBSR Intervention as an Acceptable Form of Stress Reduction

Of the 35% who dropped out, there was 31% attrition rate from the Intervention group and 38% from the control group. A total of 5 (38%) students on the 'wait-list' control group requested MBSR4 training at the end of the study. Subjective VAS levels of perceived usefulness of MBSR4 programme reported by the study completers in the intervention group were 7.4 cm (SD 2.7). The study-exit anonymous survey responses of intervention group participants are reported in Table 4. Question 1 asked about the preferred length of course, 1 participant reported the 4 weeks was the best length while the other 8 participants reported a desire for a longer course 5-8 weeks. Responses to Q2-6 are as reported.

Question 7 asked what particular part of the MBSR4 practice the students found most difficult. Six respondents consistently mentioned the difficulty of "*finding time*" to do the MBSR practice and two stated that it was also difficult to find "*a quiet place*" to practice. Question 8 asked about perceived usefulness of the programme. Responses included: *"This was very helpful" [P2]; "I really enjoyed the program and think it would be beneficial for all nursing students to have at least a taster" [P3]; "Really enjoyed the course, would have been a lot better if it could have been done earlier" [P4]; "I think possibly more of the science to why mindfulness works or what we are achieving as a result of it" [P5]; "I really enjoyed the study. I felt a learned a lot about the way in which I deal with feelings and thoughts" [P6]; "Really enjoyed it" [P7].*

Table 4. Survey questions and response data

Questions	Responses	
1. Did you think the 4 week MBSR course was long enough or would you have preferred the course to be shorter or longer in duration? Please select from the following: • *Shorter, e.g., 1 – 3 weeks* • *4 weeks was ok* • *Longer e.g., 5 – 8 weeks*	 0% 11/1% (1) 88.9% (8)	
2. Did you find the practice difficult?	YES NO	66.7% (6) 33.3% (3)
3. Did you think the learned mindfulness meditation techniques will be useful in your student nursing role?	YES NO	100% (9)
4. Should the University offer this type of stress management program as part of student support services?	YES NO	100% (9)
5. Should the University offer this program as part of the regular academic curriculum?	YES NO	88.9% (8) 11.1% (1)
6. Do you think any of the MBSR techniques you learned will be useful in your student nursing role?	YES NO	100% (9)
7. Do you think the university should offer this kind of stress-management programme as an optional student support service?	YES NO	100% (9)
8. Do you think the university should offer this kind of stress-management programme as a part of the regular academic curriculum?	YES NO	88.9% (8) 11.1% (1)

DISCUSSION

This chapter reports on a mixed methods study which attempted to assess whether completion of an MBSR4 reduced transient cardiovascular 'fight or flight' stress response in the face of a psychological stress test. The lack of difference in cardiovascular data between the two groups indicates one of two possibilities. First, it is possible that MBSR4 is not an effective intervention for reducing the 'fight or flight' response to a simulated stressor and that any perceived psychological benefits reported by the subjects did not translate into physiological changes in the HPA axis mediated cardiovascular stress response. Second, the brief MBSR4 provided insufficient time for the meditation techniques to be embedded sufficiently to translate into meaningful physiological changes in the HPA axis mediated cardiovascular stress response. An RCT in police offices using a 10-minute domestic violence simulation stress test reported a significant pre-test HR increase in the control group ($p < 0.05$) compared to the intervention group after a 4-week (16 hour) biofeedback training programme [43]. The change in HR suggests that it appears possible to develop cognitive resilience in the 'fight or flight' stress response within a relatively short period, given sufficient practice time of an appropriate technique. In our study, data were not collected on adherence to MBSR4 practice out-with the 4 hours on-site training. Therefore although participants were asked to practice for 30 minutes per day for a 4 week period (equating to 14 hours) in addition to the 4 hour onsite sessions, a 'dose-responsive' analysis was not possible.

Another possible explanation is that MBSR4 may have had an effect on the SCWT-induced stress response; however the haemodynamic changes may have been too transient or subtle to be picked up by digital autonomic blood pressure monitoring equipment. Or, that some participants in this study may already have an altered cardiovascular regulatory stress-response due to already established chronic stress syndrome [24], making transient beneficial adaption mechanisms more difficult to measure. Other studies that report intra-SWCT increases in HR ($p = <0.01$) [56], changes in low frequency components of heart rate variability (indicating sympathetic nervous system dominance) [57] and HR and SBP ($p < 0.001$) - used electrocardiograph (ECG) recordings or automated devices that collected intra-test data on a minute-by-minute basis [58]. Future studies could incorporate beat-to-beat cardiovascular measurement monitoring as a means of capturing more transient or subtle cardiovascular MBSR data. Also, global intra-test measurements could inform future study findings.

The evaluation of MBSR-mediated transient stress response resilience is an important area to investigate, primarily because MBSR is now being positioned as a key intervention to enhance the effectiveness of nurses coping with work-related stress [59]. Yet, in order to demonstrate usefulness in terms of reducing adverse physiological responses, a stress-reduction technique such as MBSR, should be able to reduce the severity of the 'fight or flight' stress response. This would lessen the risk of neuro-hormonal maladaptation associated with chronic stress states. Several studies have found the presence of one or transient stress stimuli in both the clinical and academic student nursing educational experience [60]. These include examinations and assignment stressors [61], work intensity, financial concerns [62], and lack of clinical skill competency, death of a patient, lack of support from ward staff in clinical placements [63], and time-pressure and work-life balance issues [10].

The study also aimed to identify if an MBSR4 was associated with reductions in self-reported state anxiety and mindful awareness, but found no change in either subjective parameter in either group. It is not clear why there was no effect, as an MBSR4 in post-registration nurses has previously been shown to increase relaxation, decrease emotional exhaustion and improve job satisfaction [64]. As data were not collected on adherence to practice, there was no 'dose-responsive' or degree of compliance sub-group analysis possible to determine if 'dose' of practice corresponded to any meaningful state anxiety of mindful awareness trends of change. Those who participated reported positive feeling towards the intervention, although 66% of the intervention group stated that they found the practice difficult. This may suggest higher levels of practice compliancy may be necessary, however as this was a 'real world' study, we felt that close supervision of 'dose' of practice was not practical or reflective of real-world use. Longer-term effects may have been missed, due to the shortness of the programme.

A further aim of the study was to assess the acceptability of the MBSR4 in nursing students. The high levels of participant attrition in the study (31% intervention group vs. 38% control group), lower level of post-study take-up in the wait-list control group and free textual responses about time restraints from MBSR programme completers, indicates that MBSR may only have a limited appeal in the current cohort of nursing student population. Time-pressure and difficulties in work-life balance have previously been reported in nursing students, particularly those with young children [65], and given the practice and attendance requirements involved in undertaking an MBSR programme, this finding is perhaps unsurprising. The level of attrition in our cohort was similar to that seen in other studies. A 30% attrition was reported in a study evaluating an 8-week version of the MBSR programme in nursing students.[16] One study did report a lower attrition rate of 9% in nursing students for an eight-week programme [66], however in this study all participants were given 'gifts' for participation, which may account for the higher number of completers.

It is clear from the free-textual and categorical survey data responses that many participating students perceived MBSR as being a useful tool in terms of stress-reduction. Eight week versions of the MBSR programme have been found to be effective in a range of psychological and physical chronic conditions in various populations as discussed earlier. And subjective stress-related measures reported in nursing students following an 8-week programme include anxiety ($p = 0.013$) and stress [16]. Therefore it is possible that the 4-week version in this feasibility study provided insufficient time for the practice to be embedded sufficiently to produce physiological changes alongside the subjective ones.

In summary, nursing education may be able to help students develop resilience to occupational chronic stress by providing access to a range of evidence-based stress reduction techniques. As the focus on stress and compassion in nursing becomes more recognised, it may be that future cohorts of nursing students and nurse educators will view the introduction of stress-reduction interventions such as MBSR as an increasingly important component of nursing education.

Limitations

This was a relatively small study and there is a possibility that a transient cardiovascular effect may have been missed. Nevertheless, the use of a control group allowed a comparison between the cardiovascular effects of MBSR programme participants to a psychological stress test and those who had not. This was a study designed to look at the effects of a brief (4-week) MBSR programme and it is possible that a longer programme would result in different results. This is worthy of future study. Given the study size and length, the acute (transient) self-reported measures of anxiety and mindful awareness and longer-term changes in outcomes may have been missed.

Conclusion

This chapter reported on a feasibility study which assessed the effectiveness of a brief mindfulness stress reduction training programme in providing nursing students with a useful technique for improving situational (acute) stress-response resilience and reducing anxiety. Our study findings indicate that a brief MBSR4 programme appeared to have little measurable effect on acute situational stress-response resilience in nursing students. Longer term benefits of MBSR4 are not known. Uptake of the programme was not universal and a high drop-out rate was observed. Therefore future research seeking to evaluate stress reduction coping techniques in nursing students may wish to evaluate alternative coping strategies alongside MBSR interventions. Future MBSR research could consider using psychological stress tests to assess 'dose' or practice commitment required to develop measurable cardiovascular stress resilience. In conclusion, based on the finding in this study, brief (4-week) MBSR educational training does not appear to offer a universally effective stress-resilience intervention tool for nursing students.

REFERENCES

[1] Cohen-Katz J, Wiley SD, Capuano T, Baker DM, Shapiro S. The effects of mindfulness-based stress reduction on nurse stress and burout: A quantitative and qualitative study. *Holistic Nursing Practices* 2004;302-8.

[2] Arnetz B. Psychosocial challenges facing physicians of today. *Social Science and Medicine* 2001;(52):203-13.

[3] Sharkley S, Sharples A. The impact of work-related stress on mental health teams following team-based learning on clinical risk management. *Journal of Psychiatric and Mental Health Nursing* 2003;(10):73-81.

[4] Sharkley S, Sharples A. The impact of work-related stress on mental health teams following team-based learning on clinical risk management. *Journal of Psychiatric and Mental Health Nursing* 2003;(10):73-81.

[5] Clews G. NHS stress driving up nurse sick leave levels. Nursing Times. 2008. [Online] Available at: http://www.nursingtimes.net/nursing-practice/specialisms/occupational-health/nhs-stress-driving-up-nurse-sick-leave-levels/5000401.article. Accessed 28-02-2014.

[6] Lemaire JB, Wallance JE, Lewin AM, Grood JD, Schaeffer JP. The effect of a biofeedback-based stress management tool on physician stress: a randomised controlled clinical trial. *Open Medicine* 2011;5(4):154-63.

[7] Moscaritolo LM. Intervention strategies to decrease nursing student anxiety in the clinical learning environment. *Journal of Nursing Education* 2009;48(1):17-23.

[8] Pitt V, Powis D, Lebett-Jones T, Hunter S. Factors influencing nursing students' academic and clinical performance and attrition: An integrative literature review. *Nurse Education Today* 2012;(32):903-13.

[9] Jones MC, Johnston DW. Distress, stress and coping in first-year student nurses. *Journal of Advanced Nursing* 1997;(26):475-82.

[10] Pryjmachuk S, Richards DA. Predicting stress in pre-registration nursing students. *British Journal of Health Psychology* 2007;12:125-44.

[11] Pryjmachuk S, Easton K, Littlewood A. Nurse education: factors associated with attrition. *Journal of Advanced Nursing* 2008;149-60.

[12] Lambert VA, Lambert CE, Ito M. Workplace stressor, ways of coping and demographic characteristics as predictors of physical and mental health of Japanese hospital nurses. *International Journal of Nursing Studies* 2004;41:85-97.

[13] Deary IJ, Watson R, Hogston R. A longitudinal cohort study of burnout and attrition in nursing students. *Journal of Advanced Nursing* 2003;43(1):71-81.

[14] Chan CK, So WK, Fong DY. Hong Kong Baccalaureate Nursing Students' Stress and Their Coping Strategies in Clinical Practice. *Journal of Professional Nursing* 2009;25(5):307-313.

[15] Cheung RY-M, Kit-fong T. Nursing students' anxiety and clinical performance. *Journal of Nursing Education* 2011;50(5):286-9.

[16] Beddoe AE, Murphy SO. Does mindfulness decrease stress and foster empathy among nursing students. *Journal of Nursing Education* 2004;43(7):306-10.

[17] Shirey MR. An evidence-based solution for minimizing stress and anger in nursing students. *Journal of Nursing Education* 2007;46(12):568-71.

[18] Sheilds LR. Teaching Mindfulness Techniques to Nursing Students for Stress Reduction and Self-Care. Doctor of Nursing Practice Systems Change Projects. Paper 18. 2011. Report No.: 18.

[19] McVicar A. Workplace stress in nursing: a literature review. *Journal of Advanced Nursing* 2003;44(6):633-42.

[20] Onder C, Basim N. Examination of developmental models of occupational burnout using burnout profiles of nurses. *Journal of Advanced Nursing* 2008;64(5):514-23.

[21] Glanz, K., Rimer, B.K. and Lewis, F.M. (2002). Health Behavior and Health Education. *Theory, Research and Practice*. San Fransisco: Wiley and Sons.

[22] Lupien SJ, Fiocco A, Wan N, Maheu F, Lord C, Schramek T, et al. Stress hormones and human memory function across the lifespan. *Psychoneuroendocrinology* 2005;(30):225-42.

[23] Lupien SJ, Lepage M. Stress, memory, and the hippocampus: can't live with it, can't live without it. *Behavioural Brain Research* 2001;(127):137-58.

[24] Lupien S. The long and winding road to chronic stress. *Well Stressed: Manage Stress before it Turns Toxic*. 1st ed. Ontario: Johny Wiley and Sons Canada, Ltd; 2012. p. 31-42.

[25] Maslach C, Jackson SE, Leiter MP. *Maslach Burnout Inventory Manual* 3rd Edition. Palo Alto, CA: Consulting Psychologists Press, Inc; 1996.

[26] Acharya UR, Joseph KP, Kannathal N, Lim CM, Suri JS. Heart rate variability: a review. *Medical and Biological Engineering and Computing* 2006 Dec;44(12):1031-51.

[27] Kudielka B, Bellingrath S, Hellhammer D. Cortisol in burnout and vital exhaustion. *Giornale Italiano di Medicina del Lavoro ed Ergonomia* 2006;(28):1-34.

[28] Kabat-Zinn J. Mindfulness-based interventions in context: past, present and future. *Clinical Psychology: Science and Practice* 2003;(10):144-56.

[29] Mars TS, Abbey H. Mindfulness meditation practise as a healthcare intervention: A systematic review. *International Journal of Osteopathic Medicine* 2010;(13):56-66.

[30] Irving JA, Dobkin PL, Park J. Cultivating mindfulness in health care professionals: A review of empirical studies of mindfulness-based stress reduction (MBSR). *Complementary Therapies in Clinical Practice* 2009;(15):61-6.

[31] Rosenweig S, Reibel DK, Greeson JM, Edman JS, Jasser SA, McMearty KD, et al. Mindfulness-based stress reduction is associated with improved glycemic control in type 2 diabetes mellitus: A pilot study. *Alternative Therapies* 2007;13(5):36-9.

[32] Gaylord S, Palsson O, Garland E, Faurot K, Coble R, Mann J, et al. Mindfulness training reduces the severity of irritable bowel syndrome in women: results of a randomized controlled trial. *American Journal of Gastroenterology* 2011;106(9):1678-88.

[33] Sullivan MJ, Wood L, Terry J, Brantley J, Chalres A, McGee V, et al. The Support, Education, and Research in Chronic Heart Failure Study (SEARCH): A mindfulness-based psychoeducational intervention improves depression and clincal symptoms in patients with chronic heart failure. *American Heart Journal* 2009;157(1):83-91.

[34] Robert-McComb J, Tacon A, Randolph P, Caldera Y. A pilot study to examine the effects of a mindfulness based stress reduction and relaxation program on levels of stress hormones, physical functioning and submaximal exercise responses. *Journal of Alternative and Complementary Medicine* 2004;10(5):819-27.

[35] Tacon A, McComb J, Caldera Y, Randolph P. Mindfulness meditation, anxiety reduction, and heart disease. A pilot study. *Family Community Health* 2003;(26):25-53.

[36] Holzel BK, Carmody J, Vangel M, Congleton C, Yerramsetti SM, Gard T, et al. Mindfulness practice leads to increases in regional brain gray matter density. *Psychiatry Research: Neuroimaging* 2011;(191):36-43.

[37] Centre for Mindfulness Studies. Jon Kabat-Zinn: Biographical Information. 2012. [Online}. Available at: http://www.mindfulliving programs.com/whatMBSR.php. Accessed 20/06/2014.

[38] Cotton A. Private thoughts in public spheres: issues in reflection and reflective practices in nursing. *Journal of Advanced Nursing* 2001;36(512):519.

[39] NHS Education for Scotland. Flying Start: Reflective Practice. 2012. [Online]. Available at: http://www.flyingstart.scot.nhs.uk/learning-programmes/reflective-practice/. Accessed 29/08/2014.

[40] Burnard P. *Learning Human Skills: An Experiential and Reflective Guide for Nurses and Health Care Professional.* 4th ed. Oxford: Butterworth Heinemann; 2002. p. 30-1.

[41] Kang YS, Choi SY, Rye E. The effectiveness of a stress coping program based on mindfulness meditation on the stress, anxiety and depression experienced by nursing students in Korea. *Nurse Education Today* 2009;(29):538-43.

[42] Mackenzie CS, Poulin PA, Seidman-Carlson R. A brief minfulness-based stress reduction intervention for nurses and nurse aides. *Applied Nursing Research* 2006;105-9.

[43] McCraty R, Atkinson M. Resilience training program reduces physiological and psycholigical stress in police officers. *Global Advances in Healthcare and Medicine* 2012;1(5):44-66.

[44] Kabat-Zinn J. Mindfulness-based interventions in context: past, present and future. *Clinical Psychology: Science and Practice* 2003;(10):144-56.

[45] Segal ZV, Williams JMG, Teasdale JD. Mindfulness-Based Cognitive Therapy for Depression: A New Approach to Preventing Relapse. 2nd ed. Guilford Press; 2012.

[46] Williams M, Penman D. *Mindfulness: A practical guide to finding peace in a frantic world*. Piatkus; 2011.

[47] Stein PK, Boutcher SH. Heart-rate and blood-pressure responses to speech alone compared to cognitive challenges in the Stroop task. *Perception in Motor Skills* 1993;(77):668-70.

[48] Siegrist M. Reliability of the Stroop test with single-stimulus presenation. *Perception in Motor Skills* 1995;(81):1295-8.

[49] Hoshikawa Y, Yamamoto Y. Effects of Stroop color-word conflict test on the autonomic nervous system responses. *American Journal of Physiology: Heart and Circulatory Physiology* 1997;272(3):113-21

[50] Siska E. *The Stroop Colour-Word Test in Psychology and Biomedicine. Psychosomatic Medicine* 2002;32(1):45-52.

[51] Spielberger C D, Gorsuch R L, Lushene R, Vagg P R, Jacobs G A. State-Trait Anxiety Inventory for Adults Manual, Instrument and Scoring Guide. 2nd. 1983. Mind Garden Incorporated.

[52] Carlson LE, Warren Brown K. Validation of the Mindful Attention Awareness Scale in a cancer population. *Jounral of Psychosomatic Research* 2005;(58):29-33.

[53] 1 Breivik E, Bjornsson G, Skovlund E. A comparison of pain rating scales by sampling from clinical trial data. *Clinical Journal of Pain* 2000;(16):22-8.

[54] Cork RC, Issac I, Elsharydah A, Saleeni S, Zavisca F, Alexander L. A comparison of the Verbal Rating Scale And The Visual Analogue Scale For Pain Assessment. *Internet Journal of Anesthesiology* 2004;8(1).

[55] Marazzi G, Iellamo F, Volterrani M, Lombardo M, Pelliccia F, Righi D, et al. Comparison of Microlife BP A200 Plus and Omron M6 blood pressure monitors to detect atrial fibrillation in hypertensive patients. *Advances in Therapy* 2012;29(1):64-70.

[56] Barbosa D, Prada F, Glanner M, de Toledo Nobrega O, Cordova C. Cardiovascular response to Stroop Test: Comparison between the Computerized and Verbal Tests. *Arquivos Brasileiros de Cardiologia* 2010;94(4):477-81.

[57] Delaney J, Brodie D. Effects of short-term psychological stress on the time and frequency domains of heart-rate variability. *Perceptual and Motor Skills* 2000;(91):515-24.

[58] Simoes GM, Campagnaro BP, Tonini CL, Meyrelles SS, Kuniyoshi FH, Vasquez EC. Hemodynamic Reactivity to Laboratory Stressors in Healthy Subjects: Inlfuence of Gender and Family History of

Cardiovascular Diseases. *International Journal of Medical Sciences* 2013;10(7):848-56.

[59] Smith, S. A. (2014). Mindfulness-Based Stress Reduction: An Intervention to Enhance the Effectiveness of Nurses' Coping With Work-Related Stress. *International Journal of Nursing Knowledge*. DOI: 10.1111/2047-3095.12025.

[60] Edwards D, Burnard P, Bennet K, Hebden U. A longitudinal study of stress and self-esteem in student nurses. *Nurse Education Today* 2010;(30):78-84.

[61] Evans W, Kelly B. Pre-registration diploma student nurse stress and coping measure. *Nurse Education Today* 2004;(24):473-82.

[62] Brown H, Edelmann R. Project 2000: a study of expected and experienced stressor and support reported by students and qualified nurses. *Journal of Advanced Nursing* 2000;31(4):857-64.

[63] Timmins F, Kaliszer M. Aspects of nurse education programmes that frequently cause stress to nursing students - fact-finding sample survey. *Nurse Education Today* 2002;(22):203-11.

[64] Mackenzie CS, Poulin PA, Seidman-Carlson R. A brief minfulness-based stress reduction intervention for nurses and nurse aides. *Applied Nursing Research* 2006;105-9.

[65] Kang YS, Choi SY, Rye E. The effectiveness of a stress coping program based on mindfulness meditation on the stress, anxiety and depression experienced by nursing students in Korea. *Nurse Education Today* 2009;(29):538-43.

In: Alternative Medicine ISBN: 978-1-63484-826-8
Editors: E. P. Cherniack and T. Holmes © 2016 Nova Science Publishers, Inc.

Chapter 5

THE USE OF COMPLEMENTARY AND ALTERNATIVE MEDICINES IN PSYCHIATRIC DISORDERS

David W. Thrower* and Oliver Grundmann#
Department of Medicinal Chemistry, College of Pharmacy,
University of Florida, Gainesville, FL, US

ABSTRACT

Complementary and alternative medicine (CAM) approaches are growing in popularity for the treatment of psychological conditions, particularly to supplement pharmaceutical and psychotherapeutic therapies. There is a need for better communication between the patient, physician, and alternative practitioners, as well as for physicians and pharmacists to become more informed to be able to best benefit patients choosing to employ these options and to prevent interaction effects.

Keywords: anxiety, depression, schizophrenia, bipolar disorder, massage therapy, physical activity, hydrotherapy, diet, valerian, St. John's wort, herbal medicine, S-adenosyl methionine

* Corresponding author: David W. Thrower, MS, LMT. Address: 1345 Center Drive, Room P6-20, Gainesville, FL 32610-0485. Email: David.thrower@ufl.edu. Phone: (239) 645-3585.
# PhD, MS

INTRODUCTION

To understand how complementary and alternative medicine (CAM) approaches work most effectively, it is important for a practitioner to understand the differences between the conventional (allopathic) versus the holistic model of health and disease. Fundamentally, allopathic medicine views health as the absence of any inherent major dysfunction such as a viral infection or a broken bone [1], whereas CAM practitioners view health as a perfect abstract concept of an optimal functioning organism to be striven for, but never fully attained [2]. This concept of health is characterized by perfect, efficient functioning of the physical body, complete mental clarity, and emotional balance. To make an analogy, according to Plato's theory of forms, one can cut out a piece of wood, and physically shape it like a triangle, but one can never make it a triangle. There will always be some deviation from a perfect triangle but nonetheless, the triangle exists as an abstract concept. Similarly, in complementary and alternative medicine, health is a perfect abstract concept strived for, which is not perfectly attainable. CAM practitioners will help patients strive for optimal health by concomitantly using a combination of all treatment approaches (both allopathic and CAM) available. Many modalities that support the goal of perfect health may not come in the form of a drug or a physical therapy which allopathic medicine stereotypically uses.

In integrative medicine, health, both physical and mental/spiritual is portrayed as a dimension model, where the dimensions each act as variables that contribute to the status of overall health [3]. These dimensions are (1) mechanical/physical/structural health, (2) mental/spiritual/emotional health, and (3) biochemical aspects of health [4,5]. It is generally believed that a shortfall in any of these areas will adversely affect health in all other areas to varying degrees. Conversely, improving the status of health in any of these areas will benefit the overall health of the patient. This abstract concept has been supported by many traditional medicine approaches and acknowledged to some degree by Western medicine as well. An example to illustrate the balance between these three dimensions of health is patients with moderate to severe chronic pain have an increased likelihood to experience depression [6-8]. Likewise, patients who are depressed are likely to experience pain differently from a mentally healthy person. Another observation associates cancer with not only physical pain but also depression and schizophrenia [9,10]. Those with psychiatric illnesses are more prone to diabetes, heart attack, stroke, COPD, breast cancer, colon cancer, and lung cancer [11-15]. An association has been made between type II diabetes and depression, which seemed to be linked to potential weight issues that affect both men and women. This is an example of an association between mental aspects of health and structural aspects of health. Such examples depict an association albeit not necessarily causal relationship between physical diseases and mental disorders, as well as between biochemical derangements and mental disorders. Based on this, it is viewed as ideal to address all of these areas of health concurrently in order to have the best outcome for any complaint, whether structural (e.g., arthritis), mental (e.g., depression), or biochemical (e.g., diabetes mellitus) [16]. In allopathic medicine, conditions are often segregated when they may be best addressed concurrently as Markowitz mentions regarding depressive symptoms and diabetic symptoms [16] and seen as comorbid disorders [17-19]. Many integrative techniques may benefit more than one area, such as massage therapy, which can have anxiolytic and antidepressive properties as well as benefits for structural complaints. Also, glycemic control may be beneficial to depression [20].

Overview and Classification of Treatment Interventions

Throughout this chapter, several categories of CAM treatments will be addressed for various disorders incorporating all 3 aspects of a balanced human being (i.e., mental, structural, and biochemical health). Most interventions available for the treatment of mental disorders tend to be constituents of more than one category. This list is not exhaustive but focuses on the most commonly encountered CAM approaches utilized today (Table 1).

For various clinical mental disorders and adjustment syndromes, there is a wide spectrum of treatment options which are applicable for each disorder and the severity of the condition. For example, mild dysthymic depression can be treated with massage therapy or hydrotherapy [21-23] alone, while moderate depression can be treated with St. John's Wort or 5-hydroxytryptophan (5-HTP) in addition to massage therapy [24], while others serve as adjunctive and palliative care such as use of yoga, spa hydrotherapy, and/or music therapy [25] in the management of anxiety symptoms [26-29] or depression [4,21-23,30-37]. In general, pairing all treatments with cognitive psychotherapy and other psychotherapy modalities yields the most effective long term or even permanent results. This integrative approach utilizes CAM therapies often in combination with allopathic approaches to treat the patient as a whole through physical, biochemical, and emotional care. Current research tends to support the argument that addressing all three of these areas of health concurrently typically yields more favorable outcomes [4]. An integrative approach therefore will add complexity to the treatment plan, and it becomes a cooperative effort by a team of healthcare professionals with varying professional backgrounds and levels of training including but not limited to psychiatrists, pharmacists, integrative medical doctors, and primary care providers.

Table 1. Most commonly encountered CAM approaches

Mental/Spiritual/ Emotional Interventions	Structural/Mechanical Interventions	Biochemical Interventions
Counseling	Chiropractic	Dietary Modification
Change of scenery	Physical Therapy	Herbal Medicine
Yoga		Clinical nutrition
Hydrotherapy (e.g., hot tub/percussion douche)		Vitamin and Mineral Supplementation
Meditation	Exercise	Modulation of water intake
Watsu		Colonics
Increased Social Interactions	Physical Contact	Sweat Lodge/Sauna
Massage Therapy		Aromatherapy
Hypnotherapy	Stretching	Administration of Agents that Accelerate Toxin Excretion (i.e., chelation therapy; use of naturally occurring diuretics)
Aromatherapy		

CURRENT CHALLENGES TO INTEGRATING COMPLEMENTARY AND ALTERNATIVE MEDICINE INTO MAINSTREAM PSYCHIATRY

Historically, there has been virtually no collaboration between the CAM practitioner and the primary physician in coordinating the care of the patient whether a psychiatrist, internist, or family general practitioner. Physicians are also usually unaware of their patients' use of complementary and alternative medicines [38] and are skeptical of CAM in general [39]. This problem has a twofold root. One factor is that a lot of secondary literature is skeptical of complementary and alternative medicine, including modalities that have a reasonable base of scientific support, and many physicians hold the same attitude [40]. Another is insufficient continuing education in complementary and alternative medicine. In past decades, the base of scientific evidence supporting most modalities of CAM was severely limited, but has developed and evolved since. Many practitioners may be basing their decisions on the evidence that was available at the time of their initial training, not the current state of evidence.

Communication is one of the greatest shortfalls which have encumbered the integration of complementary and alternative medicine into psychiatry. In an ideal situation, there should be a mechanism by which professionals of all modalities communicate and collaborate, so they are aware of each other's intervention plans, and can collaborate and mutually adjust their plans as necessary to achieve the best treatment outcome for the patient. There are some obvious hurdles to this especially from conventional practitioners that do not see the value in the more holistic CAM approach [3]. Though this is the case, and there is not always sufficient data to support all decisions made by some CAM practitioners, it benefits the healthcare professional and the patient to collaborate with CAM practitioners and be familiar with the known and proposed mechanisms of action of their selected therapies even when they are not fully supported, so as to be aware with what a patient is likely doing and any contraindications and special considerations related thereto. There have been many incidents caused by practitioners not being familiar with the mechanisms of action and interactions with a patient's existing CAM therapies and drugs added to their therapy [41-43]. This leads into another problem: training on the side of the attending physician and the pharmacist. Most physicians have very little training in CAM modalities [44], particularly herbal medicine, which is commonly used by patients preferring CAM. As with all drugs, herbal drugs have potential interactions, usually less pronounced than synthetic drugs, but in some cases, the interaction can present life threatening complications, such as serotonin syndrome and other complications as is the case with St. John's Wort and 5-hydroxytryptophan (5-HTP) [45-48]. An increasing number of health science colleges now offer elective courses and continuing education which can increase a practitioner's awareness and competence in this area.

This information is clearly increasingly important for all practitioner's to be trained in, as the use of CAM is on the rise. The application of conventional medicine not considering the patient's current regimen can result in duplicative therapy or serious interactions. In any case, it is crucial that if a patient is using any complementary therapy with which the physician is not familiar, that the physician must take the time to research or contact a specialist regarding whatever is being used by the patient, and hold off on making any prescription until fully aware of the risks and benefits of doing so considering their current supplements and drugs. Certain conditions such as anxiety, depression, and autism spectrum disorders may benefit at least in palliative care from a number of complementary therapies.

Sometimes abruptly withdrawing a patient from an herbal treatment may have similar risks and adverse events as withdrawing from a prescription medication. For example, withdrawing from St. John's Wort can have similar effects to withdrawing from a selective serotonin-reuptake inhibitor [49-51]. There is some evidence that a patient withdrawing from an herbal GABAergic anxiolytic such as kava or valerian may encounter similar effects [52] as one abruptly withdrawing from benzodiazepines [53] since both share similar clinical effects and a similar mechanism of action [54-60]. Likewise, withdrawing from an herbal medicine and immediately starting an incompatible prescription medication can also present with serious interaction effects, as in the case of withdrawing from St. John's Wort (monoamine oxidase and serotonin reuptake inhibitor) and immediately or within a week of cessation beginning any selective serotonin reuptake inhibitor (SSRI), tricyclic, monoamine oxidase inhibitor (MAOI), or any other serotonergic drug leading to serotonin syndrome [6]. Taking a GABAergic herbal sedative such as valerian with a drug such as a benzodiazepine can also cause interaction effects similar to those of taking two benzodiazepines concomitantly [57]. Many patients who are using these therapies and are satisfied with the results or are using supplements to complement their current treatments are often hesitant to change their treatment plans [38,61]. It is also important to note that withdrawing from a current therapy which the patient is finding effective could precipitate the patient's condition, possibly rendering it refractory to future treatment in some cases [62].

Based on this, as long as the therapies a patient is using are indicated for supportive or adjunct care of their condition, it is usually best to integrate the CAM treatments a patient is taking rather than direct them to stop taking them and use another course of treatment altogether. Using this approach may improve patient safety and patient cooperation. It is crucial that a physician presents to the patient a positive attitude toward any reasonable complementary therapies in order to attain patient cooperation and understand which supplements a patient is taking. If a physician makes a patient feel criticized after disclosing a natural treatment to them, the patient may choose not to disclose their CAM therapies in the future, possibly leading to a sentinel event due to drug-supplement interactions. This cooperation and communication ensures that decisions made are compatible with their preferred treatment and benefit the practitioner-patient relationship. Common interactions will be discussed in detail in the next section detailing intervention options in the subsection on biochemical interventions.

COMMON CAM THERAPIES AND THEIR PROPOSED MECHANISMS OF ACTION

Mental Interventions

In integrative/alternative approaches for mental interventions, modalities of psychotherapy are core, though structural and biochemical approaches are also used. There are many modalities of psychotherapy available which can be utilizes for specific disorders. These range from humanistic psychotherapy which increases a depressed patient's self-esteem to various cognitive therapy techniques which can deflate the self-esteem of someone who has a pathologically high self-esteem, for example a narcissist being treated with Festinger's approach to therapy [63]. Since psychotherapy has been a part of conventional medicine, little discussion is devoted to this topic in this chapter, however it should be noted that psychotherapy is often used in conjunction with lifestyle changes as a primary long term therapy and other supportive therapies, particularly biochemical interventions, as secondary short term treatments. This is in wide contrast to the conventional treatment mindset, where drugs are used as a primary long term course of treatment, and psychotherapy is used for short term supportive care.

General modulation of lifestyle to avoid stressors which may be contributory to one's condition may be of great benefit to many patients. Changes of scenery/entering a relaxing environment may be a good way to relieve stress for those suffering from an adjustment disorder and may be of some temporary relief for those afflicted by depression and anxiety [64, 65].

Increased social interaction is another intervention which is beneficial for those suffering from many mental conditions. A dominant variable contributing to many conditions such as major depressive disorder, generalized anxiety disorder, and social anxiety disorder is depravity of social interaction and physical contact [66, 67]. There have been several studies finding that children in their formative years who were in a deprived social environment are far more likely than the general population to experience a host of mental disorders as adults [68]. Many mental disorders also present with signs of shortfalls in social skills and eccentricities in mannerisms which make it cumbersome for the patient to develop and retain quality social contacts. In many cases, this can be overcome by training in social skills via cognitive therapy sessions to modulate social behavior and provide some relief of mental syndromes. As with all psychotherapeutic interventions, the patient needs to be willing to engage with the therapist and be self-critical in making changes.

Aromatherapy may provide some complementary relief for anxiety, depression, and other conditions [69-74]. There are several mechanisms by which this is possible. Many volatile aromatic plant extracts contain a host of volatile terpenes and other classes of compounds which have anxiolytic, antidepressant, and other psychotropic effects. For instance, lavender extracts (usually as lavender oil) have an anxiolytic effect by means of modulating voltage dependent calcium channels [75, 76] in hippocampal neurons. Notably, the structure of the compound linalool, which comprises ~25% of lavender oil [76], is structurally similar to pregabalin and may have a similar mechanism of action. Another proposed mechanism is the fact that many volatile agents produce a pleasant olfactory experience which may contribute to the anxiolytic and antidepressive effects in a temporary palliative manner. This can enhance the effect of many other modalities such as massage therapy and hydrotherapy in addition to psychopharmacotherapy.

Biofeedback is a therapy that uses external sensors and monitors to train a patient to recognize and contribute to positive changes in their autonomic nervous system and regulate heartbeat and respiration [77]. Evidence supports its complementary use in the treatment of anxiety symptoms as part of other disorders that cause anxiety such as autism and borderline personality disorder [77]. Biofeedback has also been determined to be effective in treating attention deficit hyperactivity disorder (ADHD/ADD) and may provide relief from depressive symptoms [78]. Biofeedback may also be a good option for pediatric patients who cannot tolerate SSRIs, as evidence supports the efficacy of biofeedback in treating depression and anxiety in this age group [79].

Physical Modalities

Of the physical interventions, massage therapy is one of the most common, and its use appears as a central theme in structural alternative therapies for the management of mental disorders. Use of regular massage therapy sessions has been shown to provide significant relief from symptoms of depression [30, 36, 37, 80, 81], anxiety [82, 83], borderline personality disorder [84], and many learning and autistic spectrum disorders [85, 86]. There are several known and proposed mechanisms by which massage therapy provides relief and contributes to the management of each individual disorder. The release of oxytocin resulting from sustained physical contact may have anxiolytic effects. As a result of the surge in oxytocin, there is a secondary increase in serotonin production as well as dopamine and endorphins [13, 14, 87]. This modulation of serotonin and dopamine concentrations may account for the antidepressant effects of this therapy. Since there is a considerable comorbidity between anxiety and depressive mental disorders and neuromuscular complaints [16-20] it is likely that the reduction in pain following massage therapy leads to reduced depressive and anxious tendencies. The physical derangement that leads to pain sensation also increases mental distress which is apparent in biochemical changes such as reduced serotonin levels, increased glutamate levels, and increased cortisol levels which then lead to further mental derangement such as depression and anxiety. Massage therapy also yields a release of endorphins which possess anxiolytic properties and are beneficial for those suffering from chronic pain disorders. Massage therapy has been found in one clinical trial to also reduce the symptoms of anorexia nervosa and bulimia nervosa [85]. Many cases of eating disorder symptoms associated with borderline personality disorder may benefit from intervention with massage therapy [88, 89], as well as anxiety and depressive symptoms as previously established.

As mentioned before, depravity of social interaction and physical contact is associated with an increased probability of experiencing a mental disorder. Treatments that reverse this depravity may increase the chances of symptom relief. Massage therapy is an intervention that directly intervenes to correct this depravity of physical contact.

Chiropractic intervention provides palliative relief from the neuromuscular derangements which are often comorbid with a range of mental illnesses [21, 24]. Since many psychotropic drugs also cause some neuromuscular derangements, this may be a good option as an adjunctive treatment for many patients. Chiropractic may also yield many of the same benefits attained through massage therapy. Many chiropractors also integrate massage therapy in their practices, which streamlines these treatments and provides the additive benefit of both modalities.

Exercise or modulation of physical activity habits is a great complementary therapy for many mental disorders. Many imbalances associated with depression and anxiety are associated with lack of physical activity [22]. Physical activity increases serotonin, dopamine, and norepinephrine levels in various areas of the brain, though the mechanism is not clear [90,91]. Physical activity resulted in remission for some patients with refractory depression [92]. Another proposed mechanism of action for physical activity's amelioration of depressive symptoms is a reduction of pro-inflammatory mediators including interleukins and cytokines associated with depression [13].

Hydrotherapy is a broad modality encompassing any treatment involving the application of water. One example is the hot tub/spa which is commonly used for its benefit for orthopedic and neuromuscular conditions. It has been shown to benefit mental disorders such as anxiety and depression [22, 93, 94]. It provides some temporary anxiolytic effect free of the side effects often experienced with pharmacotherapy [95]. This is important as hydrotherapy could be used on a daily basis without affecting intellectual faculties, social judgment, or physical faculties/coordination, and is furthermore unlikely to interact with most drugs. Many drug options such as benzodiazepines and barbiturates for anxiety disorders impair the faculties of the user at least to some degree, limiting their use to controlling major episodes, or when used daily will affect quality of life to a significant degree [96]. Although less pronounced, the same is true of many herbal interventions that may impair muscle control or lead to dizziness [97]. Hydrotherapy may therefore provide a more viable daily treatment option. For depressive patients using hydrotherapies, they may experience similar benefits as those from massage therapy and exercise. Ice baths are a great alternative for those who habitually self-injure although there has been no scientific publication on this topic to date. *Watsu* combines the benefits of hydrotherapy such as a hot tub with those of stretching/massage by conducting such physical treatments while in a pool/tub/natural body of water [98].

Biochemical Interventions

Dietary modulation is a central theme in both natural and conventional psychiatric interventions. There is clear evidence that various dietary insufficiencies are major contributing factors for many mental disorders [99, 100]. Based on the prior discussion of the three factor model it can be derived from an imbalanced diet which leads to biochemical derangements including but not limited to endocrine dysfunction resulting in derangement which can cause mental distress and both physical and mental chronic disorders. A few examples help to illustrate the importance of dietary deficiencies and potential interventions: insufficient intake of omega-3 fatty acids is (among many other biological and mental disorders) associated with an increased risk of developing bipolar disorder [101]. Conversely, administration of supplemental EPA/DHA (eicosapentaenoic acid and docosahexaenoic acid, essential omega-3 fatty acids) to patients suffering with bipolar disorders has been found to improve their outcomes, and in some cases patients experienced symptom remission [102, 103]. Various B vitamin deficiencies are associated with a greater incidence of schizophrenia and severe mental disorders [100]. Conversely in some clinical trials, supplementation of very large doses of B vitamins (orthomolecular medicine) has resulted in antipsychotic activity [104]. Supplementation of calcium and magnesium can be beneficial for anxiety and insomnia [100]. Identification of dietary insufficiencies and subsequent modification has in most cases the benefit of causing no harm, provides a cost-efficient way of assisting patients, and can at least complement conventional pharmacotherapeutic approaches.

Related to diet modification is sufficient fluid intake. There are several interventions which modulate water balance and enhance elimination of toxins. Mild dehydration can cause headaches, light-headedness, and electrolyte imbalances. These symptoms could exacerbate the discomfort and hence the symptoms of a depressed or anxious patient. Furthermore, it has been observed that prolonged dehydration and low fluid intake can lead to mental clouding and confusion as is the case in elderly hospitalized patients [105]. Maintaining adequate and proper water balance in a patient who is perhaps distracted by physical (pain) and mental (confusion, hallucination, personality disorders) distress or has lost the sense of thirst (e.g., Alzheimer's patients, psychotic patients, severely depressed patients) is crucial to their care [105].

Colonic hydrotherapy is another complementary approach to enhanced elimination of endogenous toxins and xenobiotics employed as a supplemental palliative therapy in the management of patients with mental disorders [94]. In this approach, the colon is repeatedly irrigated with a solution and allowed to drain with gravity. The solution is usually normal saline at approximately body temperature. This procedure is done with a control module connected with plastic tubing to an aperture inserted rectally which contains a valve and an intake and exit line. It is believed that colonic hydrotherapy prevents the reuptake of various fat-soluble endogenous toxins and xenobiotics in the colon that otherwise may irritate the nervous system and exacerbate the symptoms of a mental disorder [94]. This complementary approach remains controversial due to the potential nature of electrolyte imbalances and disruption of the endogenous bacterial microflora which may lead to intestinal dysfunction [106, 107].

Yet another approach to enhanced toxin elimination is administration of many dietary or pharmaceutical agents which enhance elimination. One example which is especially relevant in psychiatry is chelation therapy. Toxicity of heavy metals can induce anxiety and in severe cases cause psychosis such as paranoid schizophrenia and schizotypal personality disorder [108]. Even low dose chronic exposures to heavy metals have been shown to cause physical and mental disorders especially in the developing brain of children (e.g., lead, mercury, copper) [109, 110]. Though it is controversial, it may be of benefit in some cases to test for heavy metals with a challenge medium such as EDTA or DMSA (which are chemical metal chelators) and attempt a technique like chelation therapy, particularly if any heavy metals are elevated in the blood [100]. In this approach, a drug which has multiple locations with unbound electrons will chelate or form dative bonds with a heavy metal ion, displacing bonds which were previously between the heavy metal ion and an endogenous macromolecule. The heavy metal will therefore lose affinity for stationary macromolecules in the body and bind with higher affinity to the free chelating agent. The chelated heavy metal is sequestered and rendered harmless to the body and then eliminated in the urine. Supplementation of calcium, magnesium, and zinc should be considered since these ions are prone to being chelated as well resulting in a potential electrolyte imbalance. There is some risk of kidney damage with chelation therapy, particularly with EDTA, though this is lower with DMSA [111]. The decision whether to use chelation therapy should be based on the level of the insulting heavy metal, the hydration status of the individual patient, any concomitant use of pharmacotherapies, and the filtration function of the kidney.

There are a few other enhanced elimination techniques occasionally used. Saunas and sweat lodges may provide similar benefits and carry similar need for supplementation and electrolyte balance modulation requiring increased water consumption. Charcoal tablets are sometimes used to disrupt enterohepatic recirculation of organic toxins, though this has the tradeoff that nutrients, particular non-polar vitamins, are lost as well, and supplementation is necessary in most cases. Many of these enhanced elimination techniques are rarely used unless an acute toxicity with a heavy metal or other xenobiotic is apparent and requires critical care [112].

Common Mental Disorders as Described by the DSM-V with Complementary and Alternative Interventions

Based on the former discussion of the three areas that support overall well-being and an overview of various complementary and alternative medicine interventions, the focus of the remainder of this chapter will now be on commonly diagnosed mental disorders and how they can be approached using CAM therapies (Table 2). Of note, the diagnostic and statistical manual of mental disorders in its fifth revision (DSM-V) provides a more specified classification of mental disorders than can be covered here. The DSM-V classifications provided in Table 2 therefore do not reflect the specific subclassifications for each mental disorder but rather a general approach to each of them.

Table 2. Commonly diagnosed mental disorders and how they can be approached using CAM therapies

DSM-V disorder	DSM-V classifications	CAM interventions
Anxiety disorders	300.02 (F41.1)	Exercise, stretching/yoga, magnesium and calcium supplementation, aromatherapy, hydrotherapy, psychotherapy, herbal supplements (passion flower, kava, valerian, L-theanine, chamomile, lemongrass, skullcap)
Major depressive disorders	296.20 (F32.9)	Exercise, massage and hydrotherapy, psychotherapy, herbal supplements (St. John's Wort, *Rhodiola rosea*), 5-HTP, SAM-e, omega-3 fatty acids
Bipolar disorders	296.7 (F31.9)	Massage and hydrotherapy, yoga, psychotherapy, calcium and magnesium supplementation, low-dose lithium, herbal supplements (valerian), omega-3 fatty acids
Schizophrenia and Schizotypal Personality disorders	295.90 (F20.9), 301.22 (F21)	Folic acid, vitamin B12, vitamin B6, massage therapy
Other Personality disorders	301.9 (F60.9)	Omega-3 fatty acids, kava, passion flower, massage therapy, exercise
Adjustment disorders	309.9 (F43.20)	Kava, passion flower, hydrotherapy, calcium and magnesium supplementation, exercise

DISORDERS AND MANAGEMENT OPTIONS

Anxiety Disorders

For generalized anxiety disorder and other anxiety disorders, there is a wide array of complementary and alternative options. The first line intervention from complementary and alternative approaches includes a regimen of physical activity such as exercise and stretching/yoga [113]. Generally, massage therapy should also be included as part of the treatment plan, though as with any other intervention, it may not be useful for all patients, especially if physical disorders prevent effective application [114]. This will also provide rapid resolution of symptoms for many patients, and the cumulative effects of this intervention may be lasting. General lifestyle modification and reduction of exposure to psychological trigger stressors is also an inherent option. Some patients find palatable relief from chiropractic care as well. Psychotherapy should also be used extensively, and there is mounting evidence that this combination will be effective for most patients with mild to moderate and intermittent anxiety disorders [115]. A wide array of dietary deficiencies is associated with anxiety disorders. Derangements such as magnesium and calcium deficiency may cause or exacerbate anxiety, and some patients will experience a reduction in symptom severity and frequency when provided with supplemental calcium and magnesium [100]. More bioavailable forms of these minerals such as citrate salts should be considered, as their more rapid absorption may yield a more rapid response to treatment [116]. Dietary counseling in general should accompany other treatment decisions, to ensure that the patient is consuming a balanced diet. In some cases, withdrawing sugars from the patient's diet will yield some relief from anxiety disorder symptoms [117]. Hydrotherapy such as use of a spa/percussion douche may provide short term palliative relief.

When symptoms are refractory to these first line techniques, herbal anxiolytic drugs can be used in addition to mechanical interventions. Most recognized herbal anxiolytic supplements contain agents which act as agonists at $GABA_A$ receptors, resulting in an increased frequency of chloride influx. This reverses the effect of glutamate excitation which is presumed to be the primary mechanism involved in anxiety response. As with pharmacotherapy, most herbal supplements should only be used over a limited period of time to avoid dependence and potential loss of effectiveness [118].

For relief of mild anxiety symptoms, passion flower (*Passiflora incarnata*, Passifloraceae) is appropriate in most cases if not otherwise contraindicated

[97]. This is especially true in cases comorbid with mild depression, as one compound contained in passion flower is a weak monoamine oxidase inhibitor and may provide some relief from both syndromes [119]. Another advantage to passion flower is its lack of hypnotic side effects associated with many other anxiolytic treatments.

Another option which does not cause drowsiness is L-theanine present in green tea extracts [120]. Caution should be exercised not to confuse this supplement for L-threonine, an amino acid. L-theanine is a glutamate derivative which binds to glutamate receptors in the sympathetic branch of the autonomic nervous system without activating the receptor. It henceforth acts as a competitive antagonist, which blocks the excitatory neurotransmitter glutamate from binding to these receptors and activating them [121]. Because this only obstructs the excitatory effects of glutamate, which is not necessary for normal functioning outside of an anxiety response, use of L-theanine does not cause drowsiness, lack of coordination, and other impairment of cognitive faculties associated with most $GABA_A$ receptor agonists such as the primary prescription drug class of benzodiazepines used in anxiety disorders.

Kava is another anxiolytic (acting on the $GABA_A$ receptor), but may be associated with similar risks to the liver as many pharmaceutical drugs of various classes [122]. It should not be used with other hepatotoxic drugs, nor be used in conjunction with alcohol or by patients with a history of excessive alcohol consumption or impaired liver function. Several other options for herbal preparations which provide short-term anxiolytic effects are available which include valerian, chamomile, lemongrass, and skullcap. Most of these aside from L-theanine and passion flower may cause drowsiness and should not be used when driving, operating machinery, or making critical decisions [118].

Major Depressive Disorders

Many of the same interventions which are effective in providing palliative care in those with anxiety disorders will provide similar relief in patients with mild to moderate major depressive disorders. As with anxiety disorders, psychotherapeutic interventions should be employed for both conventional and CAM practices based on literature indicating higher success rates. Modulation of physical activity and dietary habits as well as structural interventions are front line complementary treatments for clinically diagnosed major depressive disorders and should be employed before any biochemical interventions such as drug or herbal therapy. Modulation of physical activity habits will be effective at providing both palliative relief and in some cases will provide long term remission [123-125]. While this is being employed, structural interventions, particularly massage therapy should be applied as well. In cases where the patient is melancholic, it may be more practical to begin treatment with the use of a passive modality of physical interventions such as massage therapy then after some relief is attained, begin initiating self-directed physical activity [80]. Hydrotherapy may provide some palliative relief, but is not likely to have any sustained improvement [93]. Nonetheless, if it is of benefit to the patient and not otherwise contraindicated, it should be considered as part of the complementary treatment approach. If the condition is refractory after a few weeks of front line therapies such as diet modification, physical activity, and physical interventions in conjunction with psychotherapy then, unless otherwise contraindicated, biochemical interventions should be implemented [126].

The use of St. John's Wort is one of the most common interventions, demonstrated more effective than placebo and non-inferior to SSRIs in the treatment of mild to moderate depressive disorders [127]. The attrition rate due to side effects is lower with St. John's Wort than with other antidepressants [128,129]. Judicious use of 5-hydroxytryptophan is another effective and safe treatment [130]. Several other interventions such as S-adenosyl methionine (SAMe) and *Rhodiola rosea* may be indicated depending on the patient's individual circumstances [131]. S-adenosyl methionine has also been found in clinical trials to be associated with statistically significant reductions in symptoms of major depressive disorder, even in patients who were previously treated with SSRIs, tricyclic antidepressants, and MAOI drugs with no response to them [132,133]. The attrition rate for SAM-e due to side effects was no more than 5% [134].

Synthetic and natural antidepressants often can interact, and simultaneous administration requires caution particularly for the risk of serotonin syndrome, which is potentially life-threatening, as a result of increased serotonin concentrations in the CNS [135]. High-dose supplementation with omega-3 fatty acids is also effective for major depression, but may not work in patients with a comorbidity of anxiety disorders [136, 137].

Bipolar Disorders

For those with bipolar disorders, there is a broad spectrum of treatment needs, as the severity of symptoms varies widely. This spectrum is represented in the Diagnostic and Statistical Manual (DSM) published by the American Psychiatric Association by three different classifications based on specific symptoms. The most severe bipolar disorder is Bipolar I and is characterized by an alternating pattern of extreme elations (commonly referred to as a manic state) and depressions in mood. This syndrome is generally also characterized by impulsive, reckless, or promiscuous behavior during elated periods. These cases are usually managed with medications including atypical antipsychotics such as aripiprazole and risperidone or agonists of the $GABA_A$ receptor such as valproic acid [138].

Some bipolar I symptoms can also benefit from dietary supplementation. For instance the mechanism of action for valerianic acid from valerian is similar to that of valproic acid and they are even structurally similar [139]. Another approach in managing Bipolar disorders with low dose lithium supplementation has been successful [140]. The dose is much lower than standard pharmacotherapy with lithium for bipolar disorders, and may be more tolerable for the patient.

Bipolar II is associated with hypomanic (elated) states without significant patterns of highly impulsive or reckless behavior and less severe elevations and depressions in behavior. These often will require similar types of treatment as bipolar I.

A third classification of bipolar disorders is cyclothymic disorder. This is associated with a continuous pattern of mild elation and dysthymia (subclinical depression). These symptoms usually do not require medication and can be managed with a combination of cognitive behavioral therapy and lifestyle changes that may include manual therapies such as massage therapy and yoga [141].

For most patients diagnosed with bipolar I, medical intervention paired with their complementary and alternative treatment is usually necessary, though some may have a significant reduction in symptoms from low-dose lithium therapy alone [142]. The sustained pattern of periods of dysthymia (mild depressive complaints) and hypomania (a mild elated state without a full manic state developing) present in cyclothymic patients may also occasionally occur in healthy individuals, but those with cyclothymic disorder are practically always in one state or the other. For these individuals, a course of complementary and alternative treatments and psychotherapy is usually sufficient. Patients with bipolar disorder II which falls between bipolar I and cyclothymic disorder in terms of symptom severity may respond to complementary and alternative treatment and psychotherapy, though many will need conventional pharmacological therapy as the fundamental therapeutic approach. As with the management of most mental illnesses, physical activity is a key element to a more holistic treatment plan [124]. In many cases, a patient will also find palliative relief from massage or hydrotherapy and other modalities of physical complementary interventions [143]. Mineral supplementation with magnesium and calcium has also demonstrated some benefits [100,144]. Dietary modification may be considered in many cases. An often successful dietary intervention is the supplemental use of omega-3 essential fatty acids. In many cases, those with bipolar disorders will find a lasting reduction in depressive symptoms after high dose supplementation of the omega-3 essential fatty acids EPA/DHA [102, 103, 145].

Schizophrenia and Schizotypal Personality Disorder

Two related disorders, paranoid schizophrenia and schizotypal personality disorder, usually require pharmacotherapy, but in many cases, using high doses of folic acid and vitamin B12 can cause a reduction in symptoms [100]. Vitamin B6 is also good as a supplemental therapy for management of both positive and negative symptoms in these patients [104]. Positive symptoms may manifest as episodes of hyperactivity, loss of connection with reality including hallucinations and delusions, and mania, whereas negative symptoms are reflected in poor social interactions, speech impediments, intermittent loss of motor control, and isolation from caregivers and social environments [146]. Careful examination of the structures of many antipsychotic drugs will reveal some similarities in their substructures which may explain their probable cross-reactivity for dopamine, norepinephrine, and epinephrine receptors [147]. Similar caution in prescribing supplements should be exercised as with prescribing conventional antipsychotics as side effects are similar including tardive dyskinesia, and even the potential for development of neuroleptic malignant syndrome based on a similar mechanism of action [148].

A central factor in utilizing complementary therapies for patients with schizophrenia and schizotypal disorders is to first achieve a state of clarity and connection with reality, which usually has to be achieved through pharmacotherapy. Such complementary therapies include diet modification, counseling, and structural interventions such as massage therapy [100,149,150].

Personality Disorders (Other Than Schizotypal Personality Disorder)

Personality disorders are among the most refractory to pharmaceutical treatment of all mental disorders [151]. In many cases a patient suffering from a personality disorder will be refractory to currently available pharmacotherapy for treatment of the primary symptoms [152]. The only supplements that have shown effectiveness are omega-3 fatty acids even as a monotherapy and even in severe cases of borderline personality disorder [153, 154]. This premise makes psychotherapy and complementary and alternative therapies the key to treating these disorders [155]. To date, only palliative and supportive treatment of symptoms is available besides long- term psychotherapy. Many personality disorders require restructuring of the patient's social environment and establishing a set of routines to manage daily life [156]. Personality disorders are also associated with considerable concomitant depressive and anxiety disorders as a result of the social stigmatization and isolation associated with the symptoms [157, 158]. Anxiolytic herbal supplements such as kava or passion flower may be useful as well as massage therapy, biofeedback, and exercise.

Cluster B (Dramatic) Personality Disorders

Though there is some evidence that atypical antipsychotic and mood stabilizers may have some benefit to those suffering from borderline personality disorder, the benefit is very minimal and usually not justified given the risks for many of these drugs [89]. In general, the front-line complementary treatment in both mainstream conventional treatments and complementary and alternative approaches is cognitive psychotherapy. Although not complementary, lifestyle modifications such as setting rigid boundaries with the patient and training the patient to set realistic expectations of others have proven effective in mitigating behavioral symptoms [159].

In patients with a disorder in this cluster, patient cooperation is usually weak, and psychotherapy and other lifestyle modifications are difficult to adhere to, but with proper modification of social structure and boundaries being set by friends and family members, this can happen. Despite limited data in regards to adherence, patients often find it easier to comply with some complementary therapies than conventional therapies based on less severe adverse effects [160, 161]. For instance, a patient convinced they do not have a problem may be more likely to cooperate with diet therapy, exercise, and massage therapy that may not appear to be directed specifically to their condition than to cooperate with a medication regimen or psychotherapy. Modulation of dietary behavior and dietary supplementation may be important as well as some conditions in this cluster are associated with lifestyle choices that may contribute to poor eating habits (frequently comorbid with eating disorders), and behaviors that cause greater nutritional needs such as alcohol abuse, drug abuse, and smoking [88]. In addition poor diet can exacerbate the anxiety and irritability associated with this condition [162, 163].

Some herbal preparations such as passion flower, valerian, kava, and other anxiolytic herbs may be of some palliative benefit to the patient, but for many of these, the medication and supplements should be managed by another party to prevent the patient from abusing them. It may be noted that in general, patients are more willing to cooperate when treated with many alternative therapies than conventional therapies due to fewer side effects. Some patients also have an unmet need and preference for direct physical interaction involved in massage therapy to establish social connections [164].

There are other cluster B (dramatic) personality disorders, such as histrionic and narcissistic personality disorders, which require less treatment and are largely controlled through psychotherapy.

Cluster C (Anxious Personality Disorders)

These disorders include obsessive-compulsive personality disorder (OCD), which is characterized by an obsession with order and routine to the degree that the associated behaviors annoy others and result in adverse social events or lead to isolation. These also include avoidance and dependent personality disorders which are characterized in overly aloof or attached behavior, respectively. These are treated in nearly the same manner as anxiety disorders (discussed above), except that anxiolytic agents presumably including anxiolytic herbs and antidepressants are not of much use other than palliative care of short-term anxiety due to adverse social consequences of the disorder. Psychotherapy is usually the prevalent treatment [165, 166]. Some anxiolytic herbal supplements such as passion flower and chamomile are more tolerable and more suitable for use over a short period of time than most pharmaceutical anxiolytics.

Adjustment Disorders

For adjustment disorders the first line treatments such as psychotherapy, physical activity [167], diet modification, hydrotherapy, and structural interventions [30, 114] are sufficient. Transient bouts of anxiety may also be ameliorated by short term use of anxiolytic herbs such as kava, skullcap, valerian, and passion flower [119]. Calcium and magnesium, as well as general multiple vitamin and mineral supplementation may be beneficial as well [100].

FUTURE DIRECTIONS

Integrative medicine is growing in popularity, necessitating physicians properly guide patients who prefer a synthesis of medical approaches. The growing demand of integrative medicine requires a change in consultation and treatment approaches to include a healthcare team with the patient at the center surrounded by general physicians, nurses, pharmacists, CAM providers, and even and especially in the case of mental disorders, their social network Although this model is not new and has been practiced by communities around the world (more so in Europe and Asia as well as in the US by osteopathic medicine schools) [168-170], it has been underutilized to benefit patients.

Another emerging responsibility of the physician is their responsibility to ensure that recommendations are compatible with the patient's current and planned use of both conventional and CAM therapies. This may at times result in temporary tensions between current best practices in conventional medicine and the less scientific nature of CAM therapies, but provides the provider with the unique perspective to empower patients to take responsibility and charge of their health. This shared responsibility opens up possibilities for steering the patient towards a complementary approach that does not interfere with current best practices while enhancing quality of life and actively involving the patient in the treatment decision. Patients with mental disorders such as depression and anxiety may feel stigmatized by society – it is important to provide such patients with active choices and involvement in their treatment to counteract social pressures and stigmas.

Peer reviewed research provides a growing amount of information which can be used to make recommendations on complementary approaches in treating mental disorders. Despite this increase in available literature, many healthcare providers remain skeptical in their approach to recommending or actively integrating CAM therapies into the treatment specifically of mental disorders [171]. The current research indicates that offering or supporting the patient's decision to use CAM therapies in addition to conventional treatments increase quality of life and treatment outcomes while lowering the total healthcare costs [169,172,173]. More research on the mechanisms of action, benefits, and risks have yet to be conducted and should be actively supported at the state, regional, federal, and international level. Identities of major active compounds for herbal supplements, a risk-to-benefit evaluation, and evaluation of potential drug interactions are also needed to increase both patient and provider confidence.

Conflict of Interest Statement

The authors declare no conflict of interest in any part of this chapter.

References

[1] Hsiao AF, Hays RD, Ryan GW et al. A Self-Report Measure of Clinicians' Orientation toward Integrative Medicine. *Health Serv Res* 2005; 40: 1553-1569.

[2] McGaghie WC. Varieties of Integrative Scholarship: Why Rules of Evidence, Criteria, and Standards Matter. *Acad Med* 2014.

[3] Chung V, Chong M, Hong LC et al. Emotionless holism: factor and Rasch analysis of the Chinese Integrative Medicine Attitude Questionnaire. *Chin J Integr Med* 2012; 18: 457-465.

[4] Thie J, Thie M. *Touch for Health. 1st ed. Camarillo*, CA: DeVorss and Company; 2012.

[5] Sutker PB, Adams HE eds. Comprehensive Handbook of Psychopathology. 3rd ed. New York: Kluwer Academic Publishers; 2002.

[6] Bair MJ, Robinson RL, Katon W et al. Depression and pain comorbidity: a literature review. *Arch Intern Med* 2003; 163: 2433-2445.

[7] Trivedi MH. The link between depression and physical symptoms. *Prim Care Companion J Clin Psychiatry* 2004; 6: 12-16.

[8] Lin EH, Katon W, Von Korff M et al. Effect of improving depression care on pain and functional outcomes among older adults with arthritis: a randomized controlled trial. *Jama* 2003; 290: 2428-2429.

[9] Hippisley-Cox J, Vinogradova Y, Coupland C et al. Risk of malignancy in patients with schizophrenia or bipolar disorder: nested case-control study. *Arch Gen Psychiatry* 2007; 64: 1368-1376.

[10] Lichtermann D, Ekelund J, Pukkala E et al. Incidence of cancer among persons with schizophrenia and their relatives. *Arch Gen Psychiatry* 2001; 58: 573-578.

[11] Mezuk B, Eaton WW, Albrecht S et al. Depression and type 2 diabetes over the lifespan: a meta-analysis. *Diabetes Care* 2008; 31: 2383-2390.

[12] Rugulies R. Depression as a predictor for coronary heart disease. a review and meta-analysis. *Am J Prev Med* 2002; 23: 51-61.

[13] Larson SL, Owens PL, Ford D et al. Depressive disorder, dysthymia, and risk of stroke: thirteen-year follow-up from the Baltimore epidemiologic catchment area study. *Stroke* 2001; 32: 1979-1983.

[14] Himelhoch S, Lehman A, Kreyenbuhl J et al. Prevalence of chronic obstructive pulmonary disease among those with serious mental illness. *Am J Psychiatry* 2004; 161: 2317-2319.

[15] Moy ML, Reilly JJ, Ries AL et al. Multivariate models of determinants of health-related quality of life in severe chronic obstructive pulmonary disease. *J Rehabil Res Dev* 2009; 46: 643-654.

[16] Rustad JK, Musselman DL, Nemeroff CB. The relationship of depression and diabetes: pathophysiological and treatment implications. *Psychoneuroendocrinology* 2011; 36: 1276-1286.

[17] Goldney RD, Phillips PJ, Fisher LJ et al. Diabetes, depression, and quality of life: a population study. *Diabetes Care* 2004; 27: 1066-1070.

[18] Roy T, Lloyd CE. Epidemiology of depression and diabetes: a systematic review. *J Affect Disord* 2012; 142 Suppl: S8-21.

[19] Goldberg D. The detection and treatment of depression in the physically ill. *World Psychiatry* 2010; 9: 16-20.

[20] Markowitz SM, Gonzalez JS, Wilkinson JL et al. A review of treating depression in diabetes: emerging findings. *Psychosomatics* 2011; 52: 1-18.

[21] Castro-Sanchez AM, Mataran-Penarrocha GA, Lara-Palomo I et al. Hydrotherapy for the treatment of pain in people with multiple sclerosis: a randomized controlled trial. *Evid Based Complement Alternat Med* 2012; 2012: 473963.
[22] Mooventhan A, Nivethitha L. Scientific evidence-based effects of hydrotherapy on various systems of the body. *N Am J Med Sci* 2014; 6: 199-209.
[23] Shevchuk NA. Adapted cold shower as a potential treatment for depression. *Med Hypotheses* 2008; 70: 995-1001.
[24] Nahas R, Sheikh O. Complementary and alternative medicine for the treatment of major depressive disorder. *Can Fam Physician* 2011; 57: 659-663.
[25] Hilliard RE. Music Therapy in Hospice and Palliative Care: a Review of the Empirical Data. *Evid Based Complement Alternat Med* 2005; 2: 173-178.
[26] Levine BA. Use of hydrotherapy in reduction of anxiety. *Psychol Rep* 1984; 55: 526.
[27] Im SH, Han EY. Improvement in anxiety and pain after whole body whirlpool hydrotherapy among patients with myofascial pain syndrome. *Ann Rehabil Med* 2013; 37: 534-540.
[28] Keegan L. Therapies to reduce stress and anxiety. *Crit Care Nurs Clin North Am* 2003; 15: 321-327.
[29] Benfield RD, Hortobagyi T, Tanner CJ et al. The effects of hydrotherapy on anxiety, pain, neuroendocrine responses, and contraction dynamics during labor. *Biol Res Nurs* 2010; 12: 28-36.
[30] Field T, Grizzle N, Scafidi F et al. Massage and relaxation therapies' effects on depressed adolescent mothers. *Adolescence* 1996; 31: 903-911.
[31] Ironson G, Field T, Scafidi F et al. Massage therapy is associated with enhancement of the immune system's cytotoxic capacity. *Int J Neurosci* 1996; 84: 205-217.
[32] Sunshine W, Field TM, Quintino O et al. Fibromyalgia benefits from massage therapy and transcutaneous electrical stimulation. *J Clin Rheumatol* 1996; 2: 18-22.
[33] Field T, Hernandez-Reif M, Taylor S et al. Labor pain is reduced by massage therapy. *J Psychosom Obstet Gynaecol* 1997; 18: 286-291.
[34] Field T, Quintino O, Henteleff T et al. Job stress reduction therapies. *Altern Ther Health Med* 1997; 3: 54-56.
[35] Field TM. Massage therapy effects. *Am Psychol* 1998; 53: 1270-1281.

[36] Lee YM. [Effect of self-foot reflexology massage on depression, stress responses and immune functions of middle aged women]. Taehan Kanho *Hakhoe Chi* 2006; 36: 179-188.

[37] Falkensteiner M, Mantovan F, Muller I et al. The use of massage therapy for reducing pain, anxiety, and depression in oncological palliative care patients: a narrative review of the literature. *ISRN Nurs* 2011; 2011: 929868.

[38] Oldendick R, Coker AL, Wieland D et al. Population-based survey of complementary and alternative medicine usage, patient satisfaction, and physician involvement. South Carolina Complementary Medicine Program Baseline Research Team. *South Med J* 2000; 93: 375-381.

[39] Hilbers J, Lewis C. Complementary health therapies: moving towards an integrated health model. *Collegian* 2013; 20: 51-60.

[40] Berman BM, Singh BK, Lao L et al. Physicians' attitudes toward complementary or alternative medicine: a regional survey. *J Am Board Fam Pract* 1995; 8: 361-366.

[41] Skovgaard L, Pedersen IK, Verhoef M. Use of bodily sensations as a risk assessment tool: exploring people with Multiple Sclerosis' views on risks of negative interactions between herbal medicine and conventional drug therapies. *BMC Complement Altern Med* 2014; 14: 59.

[42] Scarton LA, Del Fiol G, Treitler-Zeng Q. Completeness, accuracy, and presentation of information on interactions between prescription drugs and alternative medicines: an internet review. *Stud Health Technol Inform* 2013; 192: 841-845.

[43] Gilmour J, Harrison C, Asadi L et al. Natural health product-drug interactions: evolving responsibilities to take complementary and alternative medicine into account. *Pediatrics* 2011; 128 Suppl 4: S155-160.

[44] Konefal J. The challenge of educating physicians about complementary and alternative medicine. *Acad Med* 2002; 77: 847-850.

[45] Borrelli F, Izzo AA. Herb-drug interactions with St John's wort (Hypericum perforatum): an update on clinical observations. *AAPS J* 2009; 11: 710-727.

[46] Khawaja IS, Marotta RF, Lippmann S. Herbal medicines as a factor in delirium. *Psychiatr Serv* 1999; 50: 969-970.

[47] Miller LG. Herbal medicinals: selected clinical considerations focusing on known or potential drug-herb interactions. *Arch Intern Med* 1998; 158: 2200-2211.

[48] Yue QY, Bergquist C, Gerden B. Safety of St John's wort (Hypericum perforatum). *Lancet* 2000; 355: 576-577.

[49] Rahimi R, Nikfar S, Abdollahi M. Efficacy and tolerability of Hypericum perforatum in major depressive disorder in comparison with selective serotonin reuptake inhibitors: a meta-analysis. *Prog Neuropsychopharmacol Biol Psychiatry* 2009; 33: 118-127.

[50] Ditto KE. SSRI discontinuation syndrome. Awareness as an approach to prevention. *Postgrad Med* 2003; 114: 79-84.

[51] Warner CH, Bobo W, Warner C et al. Antidepressant discontinuation syndrome. *Am Fam Physician* 2006; 74: 449-456.

[52] Garges HP, Varia I, Doraiswamy PM. Cardiac complications and delirium associated with valerian root withdrawal. *Jama* 1998; 280: 1566-1567.

[53] Petursson H. The benzodiazepine withdrawal syndrome. *Addiction* 1994; 89: 1455-1459.

[54] Becker A, Felgentreff F, Schroder H et al. The anxiolytic effects of a Valerian extract is based on valerenic acid. *BMC Complement Altern* Med 2014; 14: 267.

[55] Benke D, Barberis A, Kopp S et al. GABA A receptors as in vivo substrate for the anxiolytic action of valerenic acid, a major constituent of valerian root extracts. *Neuropharmacology* 2009; 56: 174-181.

[56] Riedel E, Hansel R, Ehrke G. [Inhibition of gamma-aminobutyric acid catabolism by valerenic acid derivatives]. *Planta Med* 1982; 46: 219-220.

[57] Yuan CS, Mehendale S, Xiao Y et al. The gamma-aminobutyric acidergic effects of valerian and valerenic acid on rat brainstem neuronal activity. *Anesth Analg* 2004; 98: 353-358, table of contents.

[58] Hendriks H, Bos R, Woerdenbag HJ et al. Central nervous depressant activity of valerenic Acid in the mouse. *Planta Med* 1985; 51: 28-31.

[59] Houghton PJ. The scientific basis for the reputed activity of Valerian. *J Pharm Pharmacol* 1999; 51: 505-512.

[60] Holzgrabe U. [A riddle solved--why valerian-hops extract makes you drowsy]. *Pharm Unserer Zeit* 2004; 33: 348.

[61] Marian F, Joost K, Saini KD et al. Patient satisfaction and side effects in primary care: an observational study comparing homeopathy and conventional medicine. *BMC Complement Altern Med* 2008; 8: 52.

[62] Fauchere PA. Recurrent, persisting panic attacks after sudden discontinuation of mirtazapine treatment: A case report. *Int J Psychiatry Clin Pract* 2004; 8: 127-129.

[63] Festinger L. A *Theory of Cognitive Dissonance*. 1st ed. Stanford, CA: Stanford University Press; 1957.

[64] Schmidt CW. Environmental connections: a deeper look into mental illness. *Environ Health Perspect* 2007; 115: A404, a406-410.

[65] Rutter M. How the environment affects mental health. *Br J Psychiatry* 2005; 186: 4-6.

[66] Halls G, Cooper PJ, Creswell C. Social communication deficits: Specific associations with Social Anxiety Disorder. *J Affect Disord* 2014; 172c: 38-42.

[67] Min JA, Lee CU, Chae JH. Resilience moderates the risk of depression and anxiety symptoms on suicidal ideation in patients with depression and/or anxiety disorders. *Compr Psychiatry* 2015; 56: 103-111.

[68] McGoron L, Gleason MM, Smyke AT et al. Recovering from early deprivation: attachment mediates effects of caregiving on psychopathology. *J Am Acad Child Adolesc Psychiatry* 2012; 51: 683-693.

[69] Tang SK, Tse MY. Aromatherapy: does it help to relieve pain, depression, anxiety, and stress in community-dwelling older persons? *Biomed Res Int* 2014; 2014: 430195.

[70] Fayazi S, Babashahi M, Rezaei M. The effect of inhalation aromatherapy on anxiety level of the patients in preoperative period. Iran *J Nurs Midwifery Res* 2011; 16: 278-283.

[71] Cho MY, Min ES, Hur MH et al. Effects of aromatherapy on the anxiety, vital signs, and sleep quality of percutaneous coronary intervention patients in intensive care units. *Evid Based Complement Alternat Med* 2013; 2013: 381381.

[72] Namazi M, Amir Ali Akbari S, Mojab F et al. Aromatherapy with citrus aurantium oil and anxiety during the first stage of labor. Iran Red *Crescent Med J* 2014; 16: e18371.

[73] Conrad P, Adams C. The effects of clinical aromatherapy for anxiety and depression in the high risk postpartum woman - a pilot study. *Complement Ther Clin Pract* 2012; 18: 164-168.

[74] Kuroda K, Inoue N, Ito Y et al. Sedative effects of the jasmine tea odor and (R)-(-)-linalool, one of its major odor components, on autonomic nerve activity and mood states. *Eur J Appl Physiol* 2005; 95: 107-114.

[75] Schuwald AM, Noldner M, Wilmes T et al. Lavender oil-potent anxiolytic properties via modulating voltage dependent calcium channels. *PLoS One* 2013; 8: e59998.

[76] Umezu T, Nagano K, Ito H et al. Anticonflict effects of lavender oil and identification of its active constituents. *Pharmacol Biochem Behav* 2006; 85: 713-721.
[77] Frank DL, Khorshid L, Kiffer JF et al. Biofeedback in medicine: who, when, why and how? *Ment Health Fam Med* 2010; 7: 85-91.
[78] Siepmann M, Aykac V, Unterdorfer J et al. A pilot study on the effects of heart rate variability biofeedback in patients with depression and in healthy subjects. *Appl Psychophysiol Biofeedback* 2008; 33: 195-201.
[79] Knox M, Lentini J, Cummings T et al. Game-based biofeedback for paediatric anxiety and depression. *Ment Health Fam Med* 2011; 8: 195-203.
[80] Hou WH, Chiang PT, Hsu TY et al. Treatment effects of massage therapy in depressed people: a meta-analysis. *J Clin Psychiatry* 2010; 71: 894-901.
[81] Field T, Diego MA, Hernandez-Reif M et al. Massage therapy effects on depressed pregnant women. *J Psychosom Obstet Gynaecol* 2004; 25: 115-122.
[82] Adib-Hajbaghery M, Abasi A, Rajabi-Beheshtabad R. Whole body massage for reducing anxiety and stabilizing vital signs of patients in cardiac care unit. *Med J Islam Repub Iran* 2014; 28: 47.
[83] McPherson F, McGraw L. Treating generalized anxiety disorder using complementary and alternative medicine. *Altern Ther Health Med* 2013; 19: 45-50.
[84] Brewerton TD. Services for eating disorders: how comprehensive is comprehensive? *World Psychiatry* 2009; 8: 160-162.
[85] Hart S, Field T, Hernandez-Reif M et al. Anorexia nervosa symptoms are reduced by massage therapy. *Eat Disord* 2001; 9: 289-299.
[86] Lee MS, Kim JI, Ernst E. Massage therapy for children with autism spectrum disorders: a systematic review. *J Clin Psychiatry* 2011; 72: 406-411.
[87] Field T, Hernandez-Reif M, Diego M et al. Cortisol decreases and serotonin and dopamine increase following massage therapy. *Int J Neurosci* 2005; 115: 1397-1413.
[88] Sansone RA, Sansone LA. Personality disorders as risk factors for eating disorders: clinical implications. *Nutr Clin Pract* 2010; 25: 116-121.
[89] Dubovsky AN, Kiefer MM. Borderline personality disorder in the primary care setting. *Med Clin North Am* 2014; 98: 1049-1064.
[90] Manning JS, Jackson WC. Treating depression in primary care: initial and follow-up treatment strategies. *J Clin Psychiatry* 2015; 76: e5.

[91] Stenman E, Lilja A. Increased monoaminergic neurotransmission improves compliance with physical activity recommendations in depressed patients with fatigue. *Med Hypotheses* 2013; 80: 47-49.

[92] Mura G, Moro MF, Patten SB et al. Exercise as an add-on strategy for the treatment of major depressive disorder: a systematic review. *CNS Spectr* 2014; 19: 496-508.

[93] Latorre-Roman PA, Rentero-Blanco M, Laredo-Aguilera JA et al. Effect of a 12-day balneotherapy programme on pain, mood, sleep, and depression in healthy elderly people. *Psychogeriatrics* 2015; 15: 14-19.

[94] Shevchuk NA. Hydrotherapy as a possible neuroleptic and sedative treatment. Med Hypotheses 2008; 70: 230-238.

[95] Dubois O, Salamon R, Germain C et al. Balneotherapy versus paroxetine in the treatment of generalized anxiety disorder. *Complement Ther Med* 2010; 18: 1-7.

[96] Locke AB, Kirst N, Shultz CG. Diagnosis and management of generalized anxiety disorder and panic disorder in adults. *Am Fam Physician* 2015; 91: 617-624.

[97] Lakhan SE, Vieira KF. Nutritional and herbal supplements for anxiety and anxiety-related disorders: systematic review. *Nutr J* 2010; 9: 42.

[98] Morris DM. Aquatic rehabilitation for the treatment of neurological disorders. *J Back Musculoskelet Rehabil* 1994; 4: 297-308.

[99] Maxwell PJt, Montgomery SC, Cavallazzi R et al. What micronutrient deficiencies should be considered in distinct neurological disorders? *Curr Gastroenterol Rep* 2013; 15: 331.

[100] Zell M, Grundmann O. An orthomolecular approach to the prevention and treatment of psychiatric disorders. *Adv Mind Body Med* 2012; 26: 14-28.

[101] Balanza-Martinez V, Fries GR, Colpo GD et al. Therapeutic use of omega-3 fatty acids in bipolar disorder. *Expert Rev Neurother* 2011; 11: 1029-1047.

[102] Marangell LB, Suppes T, Ketter TA et al. Omega-3 fatty acids in bipolar disorder: clinical and research considerations. *Prostaglandins Leukot Essent Fatty Acids* 2006; 75: 315-321.

[103] Stoll AL, Severus WE, Freeman MP et al. Omega 3 fatty acids in bipolar disorder: a preliminary double-blind, placebo-controlled trial. *Arch Gen Psychiatry* 1999; 56: 407-412.

[104] Lerner V, Miodownik C, Kaptsan A et al. Vitamin B6 as add-on treatment in chronic schizophrenic and schizoaffective patients: a

double-blind, placebo-controlled study. *J Clin Psychiatry* 2002; 63: 54-58.

[105] Miller MO. Evaluation and management of delirium in hospitalized older patients. *Am Fam Physician* 2008; 78: 1265-1270.

[106] Mishori R, Otubu A, Jones AA. The dangers of colon cleansing. *J Fam Pract* 2011; 60: 454-457.

[107] Holt S. Colon cleansing perils: where's the evidence? *J Fam Pract* 2011; 60: 713.

[108] Arinola G, Idonije B, Akinlade K et al. Essential trace metals and heavy metals in newly diagnosed schizophrenic patients and those on anti-psychotic medication. *J Res Med Sci* 2010; 15: 245-249.

[109] Shailesh Kumar MV, Desiraju T. Regional alterations of brain biogenic amines and GABA/glutamate levels in rats following chronic lead exposure during neonatal development. *Arch Toxicol* 1990; 64: 305-314.

[110] Kim S, Arora M, Fernandez C et al. Lead, mercury, and cadmium exposure and attention deficit hyperactivity disorder in children. *Environ Res* 2013; 126: 105-110.

[111] Cao Y, Skaug MA, Andersen O et al. Chelation therapy in intoxications with mercury, lead and copper. *J Trace Elem Med Biol* 2015; 31: 188-192.

[112] Campbell JW, Chyka PA. Physicochemical characteristics of drugs and response to repeat-dose activated charcoal. *Am J Emerg Med* 1992; 10: 208-210.

[113] Bystritsky A, Hovav S, Sherbourne C et al. Use of complementary and alternative medicine in a large sample of anxiety patients. *Psychosomatics* 2012; 53: 266-272.

[114] Field T, Ironson G, Scafidi F et al. Massage therapy reduces anxiety and enhances EEG pattern of alertness and math computations. *Int J Neurosci* 1996; 86: 197-205.

[115] Gaudlitz K, Plag J, Dimeo F et al. Aerobic exercise training facilitates the effectiveness of cognitive behavioral therapy in panic disorder. *Depress Anxiety* 2015; 32: 221-228.

[116] Walker AF, Marakis G, Christie S et al. Mg citrate found more bioavailable than other Mg preparations in a randomised, double-blind study. *Magnes Res* 2003; 16: 183-191.

[117] Nordahl TE, Semple WE, Gross M et al. Cerebral glucose metabolic differences in patients with panic disorder. *Neuropsychopharmacology* 1990; 3: 261-272.

[118] Saeed SA, Bloch RM, Antonacci DJ. Herbal and dietary supplements for treatment of anxiety disorders. *Am Fam Physician* 2007; 76: 549-556.

[119] Sarris J, Panossian A, Schweitzer I et al. Herbal medicine for depression, anxiety and insomnia: a review of psychopharmacology and clinical evidence. *Eur Neuropsychopharmacol* 2011; 21: 841-860.

[120] Camfield DA, Stough C, Farrimond J et al. Acute effects of tea constituents L-theanine, caffeine, and epigallocatechin gallate on cognitive function and mood: a systematic review and meta-analysis. *Nutr Rev* 2014; 72: 507-522.

[121] Ritsner MS, Miodownik C, Ratner Y et al. L-theanine relieves positive, activation, and anxiety symptoms in patients with schizophrenia and schizoaffective disorder: an 8-week, randomized, double-blind, placebo-controlled, 2-center study. *J Clin Psychiatry* 2011; 72: 34-42.

[122] Teschke R, Sarris J, Schweitzer I. Kava hepatotoxicity in traditional and modern use: the presumed Pacific kava paradox hypothesis revisited. Br *J Clin Pharmacol* 2012; 73: 170-174.

[123] Eyre HA, Papps E, Baune BT. Treating depression and depression-like behavior with physical activity: an immune perspective. *Front Psychiatry* 2013; 4: 3.

[124] Ng F, Dodd S, Berk M. The effects of physical activity in the acute treatment of bipolar disorder: a pilot study. *J Affect Disord* 2007; 101: 259-262.

[125] Young SN. How to increase serotonin in the human brain without drugs. *J Psychiatry Neurosci* 2007; 32: 394-399.

[126] Cleare A, Pariante CM, Young AH et al. Evidence-based guidelines for treating depressive disorders with antidepressants: A revision of the 2008 British Association for Psychopharmacology guidelines. *J Psychopharmacol* 2015; 29: 459-525.

[127] Muller WE. Current St John's wort research from mode of action to clinical efficacy. *Pharmacol Res* 2003; 47: 101-109.

[128] Linde K, Ramirez G, Mulrow CD et al. St John's wort for depression--an overview and meta-analysis of randomised clinical trials. *Bmj* 1996; 313: 253-258.

[129] Sarris J, Fava M, Schweitzer I et al. St John's wort (Hypericum perforatum) versus sertraline and placebo in major depressive disorder: continuation data from a 26-week RCT. *Pharmacopsychiatry* 2012; 45: 275-278.

[130] Jangid P, Malik P, Singh P et al. Comparative study of efficacy of l-5-hydroxytryptophan and fluoxetine in patients presenting with first depressive episode. *Asian J Psychiatr* 2013; 6: 29-34.

[131] Darbinyan V, Aslanyan G, Amroyan E et al. Clinical trial of Rhodiola rosea L. extract SHR-5 in the treatment of mild to moderate depression. *Nord J Psychiatry* 2007; 61: 343-348.

[132] Bell KM, Plon L, Bunney WE, Jr. et al. S-adenosylmethionine treatment of depression: a controlled clinical trial. *Am J Psychiatry* 1988; 145: 1110-1114.

[133] Williams AL, Girard C, Jui D et al. S-adenosylmethionine (SAMe) as treatment for depression: a systematic review. *Clin Invest Med* 2005; 28: 132-139.

[134] Kagan BL, Sultzer DL, Rosenlicht N et al. Oral S-adenosylmethionine in depression: a randomized, double-blind, placebo-controlled trial. *Am J Psychiatry* 1990; 147: 591-595.

[135] Park SH, Wackernah RC, Stimmel GL. Serotonin syndrome: is it a reason to avoid the use of tramadol with antidepressants? *J Pharm Pract* 2014; 27: 71-78.

[136] Lesperance F, Frasure-Smith N, St-Andre E et al. The efficacy of omega-3 supplementation for major depression: a randomized controlled trial. *J Clin Psychiatry* 2011; 72: 1054-1062.

[137] Osher Y, Belmaker RH. Omega-3 fatty acids in depression: a review of three studies. *CNS Neurosci Ther* 2009; 15: 128-133.

[138] Woo YS, Bahk WM, Jung YE et al. One-year rehospitalization rates of patients with first-episode bipolar mania receiving lithium or valproate and adjunctive atypical antipsychotics. *Psychiatry Clin Neurosci* 2014; 68: 418-424.

[139] Eadie MJ. Could valerian have been the first anticonvulsant? *Epilepsia* 2004; 45: 1338-1343.

[140] Sylvia LG, Reilly-Harrington NA, Leon AC et al. Methods to limit attrition in longitudinal comparative effectiveness trials: lessons from the Lithium Treatment - Moderate dose Use Study (LiTMUS) for bipolar disorder. *Clin Trials* 2012; 9: 94-101.

[141] Kemper KJ, Shannon S. Complementary and alternative medicine therapies to promote healthy moods. *Pediatr Clin North Am* 2007; 54: 901-926; x.

[142] Oruch R, Elderbi MA, Khattab HA et al. Lithium: a review of pharmacology, clinical uses, and toxicity. *Eur J Pharmacol* 2014; 740: 464-473

[143] Andreescu C, Mulsant BH, Emanuel JE. Complementary and alternative medicine in the treatment of bipolar disorder--a review of the evidence. *J Affect Disord* 2008; 110: 16-26.

[144] Sarris J, Lake J, Hoenders R. Bipolar disorder and complementary medicine: current evidence, safety issues, and clinical considerations. *J Altern Complement Med* 2011; 17: 881-890.

[145] Freeman MP, Hibbeln JR, Wisner KL et al. Omega-3 fatty acids: evidence basis for treatment and future research in psychiatry. *J Clin Psychiatry* 2006; 67: 1954-1967.

[146] Brosey E, Woodward ND. Schizotypy and clinical symptoms, cognitive function, and quality of life in individuals with a psychotic disorder. *Schizophr Res* 2015.

[147] Bender A, Scheiber J, Glick M et al. Analysis of pharmacology data and the prediction of adverse drug reactions and off-target effects from chemical structure. *Chem Med Chem* 2007; 2: 861-873.

[148] Pelonero AL, Levenson JL, Pandurangi AK. Neuroleptic malignant syndrome: a review. *Psychiatr Serv* 1998; 49: 1163-1172.

[149] Edge J. A pilot study addressing the effect of aromatherapy massage on mood, anxiety and relaxation in adult mental health. *Complement Ther Nurs Midwifery* 2003; 9: 90-97.

[150] Vancampfort D, Probst M, Knapen J et al. [Body-directed techniques on psychomotor therapy for people with schizophrenia: a review of the literature]. *Tijdschr Psychiatr* 2011; 53: 531-541.

[151] Lana F, Fernandez-San Martin MI. To what extent are specific psychotherapies for borderline personality disorders efficacious? A systematic review of published randomised controlled trials. *Actas Esp Psiquiatr* 2013; 41: 242-252.

[152] Ripoll LH. Psychopharmacologic treatment of borderline personality disorder. *Dialogues Clin Neurosci 2013*; 15: 213-224.

[153] Zanarini MC, Frankenburg FR. omega-3 Fatty acid treatment of women with borderline personality disorder: a double-blind, placebo-controlled pilot study. *Am J Psychiatry* 2003; 160: 167-169.

[154] Amminger GP, Chanen AM, Ohmann S et al. Omega-3 fatty acid supplementation in adolescents with borderline personality disorder and ultra-high risk criteria for psychosis: a post hoc subgroup analysis of a double-blind, randomized controlled trial. *Can J Psychiatry* 2013; 58: 402-408.

[155] Tyrer P, Silk KR. A comparison of UK and US guidelines for drug treatment in borderline personality disorder. *Int Rev Psychiatry* 2011; 23: 388-394.
[156] Spencer SJ, Rutter D, Tyrer P. Integration of nidotherapy into the management of mental illness and antisocial personality: a qualitative study. *Int J Soc Psychiatry* 2010; 56: 50-59.
[157] Watson D, Naragon-Gainey K. Personality, Emotions, and the Emotional Disorders. *Clin Psychol Sci* 2014; 2: 422-442.
[158] Skodol AE, Geier T, Grant BF et al. Personality disorders and the persistence of anxiety disorders in a nationally representative sample. *Depress Anxiety* 2014; 31: 721-728.
[159] Renner F, van Goor M, Huibers M et al. Short-term group schema cognitive-behavioral therapy for young adults with personality disorders and personality disorder features: associations with changes in symptomatic distress, schemas, schema modes and coping styles. *Behav Res Ther* 2013; 51: 487-492.
[160] Dimaggio G, Livesley J. Introduction to the special feature on the integrated treatment of personality disorder. *J Pers Disord* 2012; 26: 1-6.
[161] Davidson JR, Rampes H, Eisen M et al. Psychiatric disorders in primary care patients receiving complementary medical treatments. *Compr Psychiatry* 1998; 39: 16-20.
[162] Buydens-Branchey L, Branchey M, Hibbeln JR. Associations between increases in plasma n-3 polyunsaturated fatty acids following supplementation and decreases in anger and anxiety in substance abusers. *Prog Neuropsychopharmacol Biol Psychiatry* 2008; 32: 568-575.
[163] Testa A, Giannuzzi R, Sollazzo F et al. Psychiatric emergencies (part II): psychiatric disorders coexisting with organic diseases. *Eur Rev Med Pharmacol Sci* 2013; 17 Suppl 1: 65-85.
[164] Honda K, Jacobson JS. Use of complementary and alternative medicine among United States adults: the influences of personality, coping strategies, and social support. *Prev Med* 2005; 40: 46-53.
[165] Lazar SG. The cost-effectiveness of psychotherapy for the major psychiatric diagnoses. *Psychodyn Psychiatry* 2014; 42: 423-457.
[166] Leichsenring F, Salzer S. A unified protocol for the transdiagnostic psychodynamic treatment of anxiety disorders: an evidence-based approach. *Psychotherapy* (Chic) 2014; 51: 224-245.
[167] Yang X, Telama R, Hirvensalo M et al. Moderating effects of leisure-time physical activity on the association between job strain and

depressive symptoms: the Cardiovascular Risk in Young Finns Study. *J Occup Environ Med* 2012; 54: 303-309.

[168] Conrad K, Spano M, Seidman MD. Complementary and integrative treatments: healthy living: strategies to live longer. *Otolaryngol Clin North Am* 2013; 46: 277-294.

[169] Herman PM. Evaluating the economics of complementary and integrative medicine. *Glob Adv Health Med* 2013; 2: 56-63.

[170] Sun XG, Wu WK, Lu ZP. Chinese integrative medicine: translation toward person-centered and balanced medicine. *Chin J Integr Med* 2012; 18: 3-6.

[171] Cowan RP. CAM in the real world: you may practice evidence-based medicine, but your patients don't. *Headache* 2014; 54: 1097-1102.

[172] Diehl V. The bridge between patient and doctor: the shift from CAM to integrative medicine. *Hematology Am Soc Hematol Educ Program* 2009: 320-325.

[173] Maizes V, Rakel D, Niemiec C. Integrative medicine and patient-centered care. *Explore (NY)* 2009; 5: 277-289.

In: Alternative Medicine ISBN: 978-1-63484-826-8
Editors: E. P. Cherniack and T. Holmes

Chapter 6

COMPLEMENTARY AND ALTERNATIVE MEDICINE FOR PAIN MANAGEMENT

D. Priyamka Sreekeesoon and M. Fawzi Mahomoodally*

Department of Health Sciences, Faculty of Science,
University of Mauritius, Réduit, Mauritius

ABSTRACT

Pain essentially is a mere sensation which acts as herald of danger to the body, nonetheless once pain transcends the prognosis stage, it becomes no less than an ordeal resulting in repercussions including anxiety, depression, sleep disturbances, amongst others on patients' daily life. Such is the intricacy of pain that the contribution of conventional medicine in its relief despite conspicuous yet remains below par as far as management of arthritis pain, diabetic neuropathy, cancer pain, fibromyalgia, and other related conditions are concerned wherein substantial pain is endured by patients. Accordingly, due to particular constraints of mainstream medicine, there has been the resurgence and extensive use of alternative medicine in current years endorsed by ever mounting evidence of its efficacy. The success of alternative medicine has been irrefutable and momentous in alleviating chronic pain

* Corresponding author: M. Fawzi Mahomoodally, PhD. Department of Health Sciences, Faculty of Science, University of Mauritius, 230 Réduit, Mauritius. Tel.: +230 4037578; Fax: +230 4656928; E-mail: f.mahomoodally@uom.ac.mu.

conditions. This chapter attempts to overview pain and its physiology, the role of inflammation in pain perception, the classification of pain, pain assessment tools, common chronic pain conditions, widespread alternative therapies used for pain management and specific challenges of alternative medicine.

INTRODUCTION

Pain is an undesirable but essential manifestation that forewarns the body about potentially deleterious stimuli and accordingly ensures its protection (Da Silva et al. 2012). This concept underlines the biological significance of pain, which is apt in the case of acute pain as it is of short duration and generally linked to disease or injury. However, once pain lasts beyond the anticipated prognosis, in chronic or persistent pain conditions, it no longer performs its role as a herald of impeding danger (Huguet et al. 2010). When pain transcends an expected duration, it becomes an ordeal with repercussions such as anxiety, depression and sleep disturbances, that impact patients' daily life (Sprintz et al. 2011).

The International Association for the Study of Pain (IASP, 2012) defines pain as 'an unpleasant sensory and emotional experience associated with actual or potential tissue damage, or described in terms of such damage.' This definition endorses the complexity and multifariousness of pain and emphasises that pain need not necessarily involve any pathophysiological cause, but may be of psychological origin. Pain can thus be described as a sheer individualistic and singular experience that can be challenging to evaluate (Steeds, 2009) and results from the interplay of sensory, physiological, cognitive, affective, behavioural and spiritual factors (WHO, 2012).

Such is the intricacy of pain that the contribution of conventional medicine, in its potential to offer relief, despite being conspicuous, as yet remains below par, particularly in the management of arthritis pain, diabetic neuropathy, cancer pain, fibromyalgia, and other conditions wherein substantial pain is endured by patients (Turk et al. 2011; Bashir and Colvin, 2012). Due to particular constraints of mainstream medicine, there has been a resurgence and extensive use of alternative medicine in current years, endorsed by ever-mounting evidence of efficacy (Berman et al. 2009; Bruckenthal, 2010; Rehberg, 2010; Fouladbakhsh et al. 2011; Peleg et al.

2011; Yoon and Kim, 2013). The success of alternative medicine is irrefutable and momentous in alleviating chronic pain conditions.

This chapter commences with an overview of pain and its physiology, the role of inflammation in pain perception, the classification of pain, pain assessment tools, and common chronic pain conditions. It then documents widespread alternative therapies used for pain management, and discusses specific challenges of alternative medicine. The island of Mauritius is renowned for its singular biodiversity, and the use of alternative medicine is a common practice among Mauritians. A résumé of a study conducted in the island is also outlined in this chapter, highlighting commonly used alternative therapies including herbal remedies, Ayurvedic medicine, massage and yoga, reportedly influential in pain management.

The Perception of Pain

The inborn capacity to perceive pain, or 'nociception,' follows the stimulation of nociceptors which are sensory receptors, specifically unspecialized nerve cell endings located peripherally in tissues that initiate the sensation of pain. When activated by injurious or painful stimuli, nociceptors transduce the information received into electrical signals and transmit it along axons from the periphery to the central nervous system where control from higher centres occurs. The entire signal transduction pathway involved in relaying pain messages to the brain is highly complex, with involvement of the spinal cord, thalamus, cortex and midbrain (Steeds, 2009). When associated with a particular stimulus, pain can be depicted as a physiological occurrence that activates reflex withdrawal mechanisms, consequently minimising tissue injury and promoting healing (Driessen, 2007).

Inflammation and Pain

In most cases, pain is generated by inflammation, and is one of the foremost characteristics of inflammation. Arachidonic acid metabolism and the release of other pain generating substances from damaged tissues are responsible for pain trigger in an inflamed tissue. Inflammation and pain may be linked by cyclooxygenase (COX) enzymes particularly, COX_2. COX_2 helps in the synthesis of prostaglandins (PGs) in particular; PGE_2 and $PGF_{2\alpha}$which are available in high levels at the site of inflammation. The released PGs either activate pain receptor or sensitise pain receptors to the action of other pain producing substances such as histamine, 5-hydroxytryptamine (5HT), and bradykinin. This in turn activates and triggers the nerve cells to send electrical pain impulses to the brain (Arome et al. 2014).

CLASSIFICATION OF PAIN

A number of classification systems have been proposed, although as yet none are internationally recognised or accepted (WHO, 2012). The IASP has attempted to classify chronic pain according to the various body sites (IASP, 2012) but as such no classification encompasses pain as a whole. Nonetheless, a WHO publication based on guidelines for pharmacological treatment of continuous pain in children with medical illnesses shortlists four of the most utilised categories of pain, as follows:

Table 1. Common categories of pain (WHO, 2012)

Pain category	Sub-types	Description
The patho-physiological mechanism of pain	Nociceptive or neuropathic pain	Nociceptive pain occurs following the activation of nociceptors when triggered by various stimuli. Based on the location of nociceptors, it may be categorised as somatic and/or visceral pain. When nerve fibres in the peripheral or central nervous system are damaged, neuropathic pain results. This can occur due to a number of factors including pathological conditions.
The duration of pain	Chronic or acute, breakthrough pain	Acute pain usually occurs unexpectedly as a result of injury, is intense but of short duration. It involves activation of nociceptors and thus injury healing ultimately takes place. Chronic pain is persistent and lasts beyond the anticipated healing process. Chronic pain onset may be without any particular pathophysiology or medical illness.
The aetiology	Malignant or non-malignant	Whether the underlying disease is malignant or non-malignant.
The anatomic location of pain		By body location such as, head, back or neck or by anatomic functions of the affected tissue, such as myofascial, rheumatic, skeletal or neurological.

Pain Assessment

Reliable and accurate pain assessment techniques are mandatory for effective management of pain. Manifold pain assessment tools have been devised in an attempt to evaluate the intensity and duration of pain. Pain assessment apparently depends on age as the methods to evaluate pain differ for children and adults (Powell et al. 2010). The key and commonly used tools for evaluating pain in adults are illustrated below:

Table 2. Adult pain assessment tools, (Powell et al. 2010)

Scales	Descriptions
Visual analogue scale (VAS) 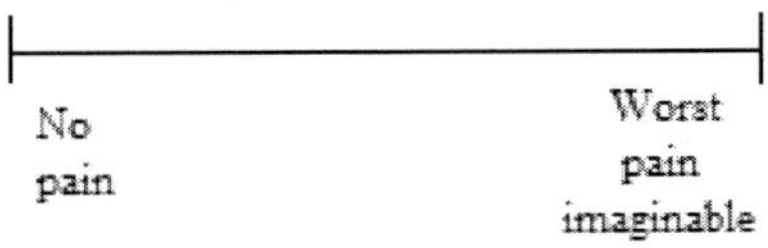	This scale uses a horizontal line, 10 cm in length, with the descriptors "No pain" and "Worst pain imaginable'' at both ends. Patients can thus indicate what best symbolises the severity of their actual pain.
Numerical rating scale 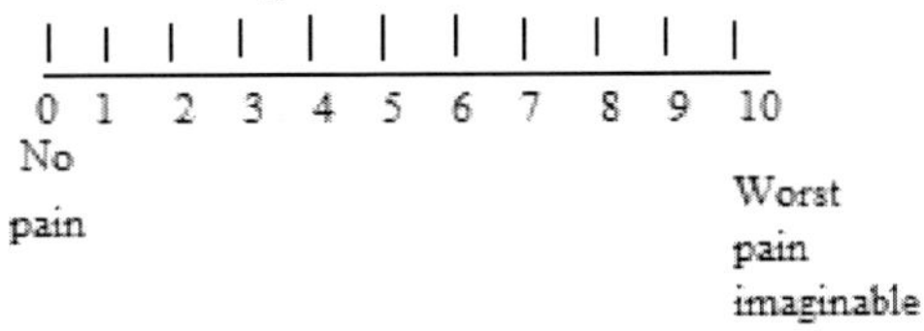	Patients can rate pain intensity on this scale which usually ranges from 0 (indicating "No pain") to 10 (indicating the "Worst pain imaginable").
Verbal descriptor scale 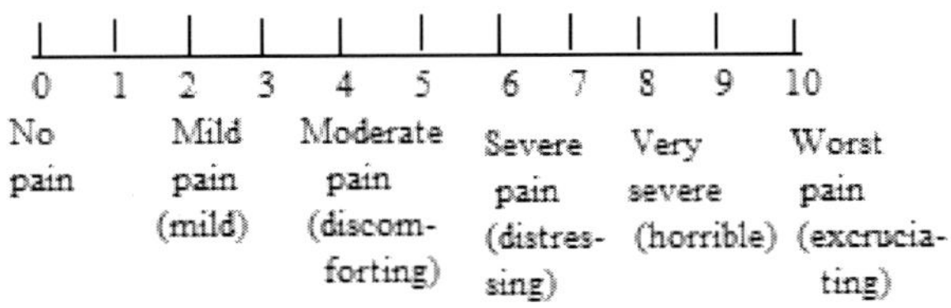	Following a description of the different pain experiences which could be felt by the patient, the health provider asks the patient to verbally or visually choose one of the following six descriptors: "No pain," "Mild pain," "Moderate pain," "Severe pain," "Very severe pain," and "Worst pain possible'', to best signify his level of pain intensity.

Pain and Related Disorders

Pain being a highly individualistic phenomenon can be complex to evaluate and treat, particularly in the majority of elderly who live with serious ailments and experience considerable pain as a symptom (Tracy and Morrison, 2013). Chronic pain in particular impacts on all aspects of daily life with distressing repercussions on health and quality of life (Fouladbakhsh et al. 2011). Widespread chronic pain conditions include low-back pain, headache, arthritis pain, pain from nerve damage (e.g., diabetic neuropathy), cancer pain, and other conditions, such as fibromyalgia, in which considerable pain is experienced (NCCAM, 2011). Some of these prevalent chronic pain syndromes are briefly reviewed here:

Musculoskeletal Disease

Musculoskeletal diseases are widespread and result in impairment and handicap impacting tremendously on the social, labour, economic and quality of life of patients and their family environment (Alfaro et al. 2013). Rheumatic diseases include more than 150 diverse conditions and syndromes and are commonly characterised by being pain and inflammation. Five of the most prevalent painful musculoskeletal conditions are: osteoarthritis, rheumatoid arthritis (RA), fibromyalgia, systemic lupus erythematosus (SLE) and gout (Vitetta et al. 2008). Arthritis is reportedly the most prevalent musculoskeletal disease, with osteoarthritis being the most common type, usually affecting the knees, hands, feet, hips, and spine (Allen and Nelson, 2013).

Fibromyalgia

Fibromyalgia is a clinical syndrome characterised by chronic widespread muscle pain, fatigue and tenderness, with unusually high sensitivity to pressure over tender points and this has severe repercussions on the daily life of patients (Dailey et al. 2013). Other symptoms such as sleep disorders, cognitive dysfunction, irritable bowel and bladder, headache, and a variety of somatic complaints can also result (Terhorst et al. 2011).

Back pain

Back pain generally has no common cause and includes a cluster of conditions. Consequently there is no standard treatment. Back pain is burdensome to patients' life quality and has dire impacts on daily life (Aickin et al. 2013).

Sciatica

Sciatica or lumbosacral radicular syndrome, particularly if resulting from lumbar intervertebral disc herniation, is amongst the most prevalent causes of radicular pain. Treatment in individuals differs considerably with some requiring spinal surgery and others reliant on non-surgical therapies. However, in recent years, little satisfaction and improvement has been reported in patients undergoing lumbar disc surgery (Edwards et al. 2007; El Barzouhi et al. 2014).

PAIN MANAGEMENT AND/OR TREATMENT

The significance of pharmacological agents including paracetamol, NSAIDs, opioids, antidepressants, anticonvulsants, skeletal muscle relaxants and topical agents cannot be contested, particularly in management of chronic pain conditions (Turk et al. 2011; Bashir and Colvin, 2012; Schofield, 2012). Furthermore, interventional pain medicine is used frequently when the pain site is located in a specific area of the spine, in which case various techniques, for instance, injection therapy, surgery and implantable devices can be adopted. Physical, rehabilitative, and psychological approaches may also be additionally used (Turk et al. 2011).

Pain management in the elderly is arduous and often leads to inadequate results. Older people may experience difficulty communicating with medical practitioners, which potentially contributes to biased treatment and prescriptions of drugs (Schofield, 2012). They may also have reduced functional status and physiological reserve, such as pharmacodynamic and pharmacokinetic alterations in renal function and hepatic metabolism, or central nervous system disorders such as dementia (Tracy and Morrison, 2013).

Furthermore, conventional therapies have specific limitations including restricted long-term effectiveness, due to tolerance issues and side effects. Consequently there is a growing interest in complementary approaches (Verkamp et al. 2013). A wealth of published studies (Berman et al. 2009; Bruckenthal, 2010; Rehberg, 2010; Fouladbakhsh et al. 2011; Peleg et al. 2011; Yoon and Kim, 2013) provide evidence regarding the escalating prevalence of complementary and alternative medicine (CAM), both self-prescribed and practitioner-administered, for pain management.

Complementary and Alternative Medicine

The National Centre for Complementary and Alternative Medicine (NCCAM) defines CAM 'as a group of diverse medical and health care interventions, practices, products, or disciplines that are not generally considered part of conventional medicine.' CAM practices can be broadly categorised as natural products, mind and body medicine, and manipulative and body-based practices with possible overlap between therapies (NCCAM, 2012).

CAM is increasingly being used for diverse pain conditions as innumerable studies have reported, including for back pain (Poole et al. 2007; Gagnier, 2008; Kirby et al. 2013; Murthy et al. 2014), fibromyalgia (Terhorst et al. 2011), labour pain (Tournaire and Theau-Yonneau, 2007; Arendt and Tessmer-Tuck, 2013), chronic pelvic pain (Paiva and Carneiro, 2013), musculoskeletal conditions (Vitetta et al. 2008), migraine (Gantenbein et al. 2012), pain in sickle cell anaemia (Majumdar et al. 2013), neck pain (Plastaras et al. 2011) among others. The most prevalent CAM for pain management will be briefly explored below:

Acupuncture

Coined in the 1600s by Jesuit missionaries, the term acupuncture is derived from the Latin *Acus* (needle) and *Puncture* (puncture), who based their observations on this healing traditionally originating from China (Dorsher, 2011). Acupuncture initially had the intricate purpose of modulating the body's imbalance of the cosmic energy, 'Yin and Yang' and it implicates the insertion of needles in specific acupuncture points on the body surface to provide a desired curative effect. Fascinatingly enough, insertion points are alongside meridians through which the vital life energy, 'Qi' flows. Following the insertion of needles, a peculiar feeling called *De qi* is experienced, which can be pain, numbness, heat, weight, or distension and this is generally desirable for effective acupuncture (Grillo et al. 2013; Peacock, 2013).

The pain-relieving effect provided by acupuncture is claimed to arise due to release of spinal dynorphin and encephalin, which are inhibitory pain neurotransmitters, through increased local blood flow and from the relaxation of muscle fibres (Peacock, 2013). Accordingly, acupuncture was found to be effective in symptomatic relief of dental pain, and it overshadows the side effects occurring with conventional pain-relieving medications, including stomach ulcers and bleeding problems. Additionally, acupuncture has numerous benefits, it is a natural, low-cost therapy and can be considered a safe procedure when conducted appropriately by a trained professional (Grillo et al. 2013).

Moxibustion

Moxibustion is a technique involving thermal stimulation by burning herbs, particularly, *Artemisia vulgaris*, by placing a small disposable moxibustion device at specific acupuncture points on the skin (Lee et al. 2013). Single or combination moxibustion therapies are shown to diminish symptoms of pain in peripheral knee osteoarthritis (Ren et al. 2012; Lee et al. 2013).

Guided Imagery

In guided imagery, as the name distinctly suggests, specific images in part or whole are instructed to patients to attain a particular therapeutic purpose (Lewandowski and Jacobson, 2013). The creation or recollection of a medley of mental images, such as perception of objects or events, engages the cognitive intellect, memory, emotional and motor control mechanisms. Images are visualized by patients in a state of relaxation, apparently with a specific outcome in mind, for instance, pain relief (Posadzki et al. 2012). Guided imagery is widespread as a complementary therapy and has been demonstrated to relieve chronic non-cancer pain (Lewandowski and Jacobson, 2013).

Herbal Remedies

Medicinal plants and their derivatives have demonstrated their worth for years as promising resources for a panoply of pharmacological agents and herbals used in pain management (Da Silva et al. 2012). Consequently, herbal analgesics can be effective in improving the quality of life of patients concurrently with conventional pain-relieving therapies. Herbal medicines have been used in a cluster of pain-related diseases including rheumatologic diseases, back pain, cancer, diabetic peripheral neuropathy and migraines (Zareba, 2009, Gagnier, 2008).

It should be highlighted that allopathic medications used for neuropathic pain are associated with various adverse effects, withdrawal syndromes, and multiple pathological mechanisms, and cannot be applied for all types of neuropathy (Muthuraman and Singh, 2012). Several publications (Wirth, 2005; Agunu et al. 2009; Zareba, 2009) describe herbal therapies used traditionally for pain management. The following table depicts prevalent medicinal plants and their purported traditional uses in pain-related conditions:

Table 3. Medicinal plants, purported traditional uses in pain-related conditions

Plants (Family)	Method of preparation/Mode of administration	Parts used	Pain-related conditions	References
Acer monspessulanum L. (Aceraceae)	Concentrated decoction with Fraxinus leaves	Aerial part	Foot pain	Mosaddegh et al. 2012
Albizia grandibracteata Taub (Fabaceae)	Decoction	Leaves	Back pain	Lacroix et al. 2011
Aubrieta parviflora Boiss (Brassicaceae)	Concentrated decoction mixed with other plants as liniment.	Aerial part	Muscle, back and foot pains	Mosaddegh et al. 2012
Chenopodium ambrosioides L. (Chenopodioideae)	Infusion/Oral	Leaves	Abdominal pain	Juárez-Vázquez et al. 2013
Glycyrrhiza glabra L. (Fabaceae)	Fresh leaf is put on the aching point; concentrated decoction of root is applied as liniment on the aching point; cooked roots.	Leaf and root	Body pains	Mosaddegh et al. 2012

Plants (Family)	Method of preparation/Mode of administration	Parts used	Pain-related conditions	References
Matricaria recutita L. (Asteraceae)	Infusion/Oral	Leaves/Whole plant	Headache, Stomach ache	Juárez-Vázquez et al. 2013
Mentha piperita L. (Lamiaceae)	Infusion/Oral	Leaves/Whole plant	Stomach ache, Headache	Juárez-Vázquez et al. 2013
Pavetta crassipes K. (Rubiaceae)	Hot water extract taken oral, one glass is taken 3 times daily for 14 days or until patient recovers.	Leaves	Chronic joint pain	Wambugu et al. 2011
Piper auritum (Piperaceae)	Infusion/Oral	Leaves/ Whole plant	Headache, Stomach ache	Juárez-Vázquez et al. 2013
Psidium guajava L. (Myrtaceae)	Infusion/Oral	Leaves	Stomach ache	Gutiérrez et al. 2008 Juárez-Vázquez et al. 2013
Ruta chalepensis L. (Rutaceae)	Infusion/Oral Infusion/Topical	Whole plant	Headache, Stomach ache	Juárez-Vázquez et al. 2013
Strychnos henningsii Gilg (Loganiaceae)	Hot water extract taken orally, one glass taken 2–3 times daily for 14 days or until patient recovers.	Leaves, stem bark	Chronic joint pain	Wambugu et al. 2011
Tagetes erecta L. (Asteraceae)	Infusion/Oral	Flower	Stomach ache	Juárez-Vázquez et al. 2013
Tagetes minuta L. (Asteraceae)	Leaves and flowers rubbed on the head	Leaves and flowers	Headache, pain	Lacroix et al. 2011
Urginea maritime (Liliaceae)	Heated bulb is put on aching tooth, Fresh bulb squashed and put around aching organ	Bulb	Tooth ache, rheumatism, joint pains	Mosaddegh et al. 2012

The analgesic, anti-nociceptive properties and efficacy of some common medicinal plants investigated in pre-clinical studies are briefly overviewed below:

Table 4. Reported analgesic and anti-nociceptive plant properties investigated in clinical studies

Medicinal plants	Endorsing *in vivo* studies	References
Acorus calamus L.	Hydro-alcoholic extract of the plant diminished vincristine induced painful neuropathy resulting possibly from its anti-oxidative, anti-inflammatory, and calcium inhibitory actions.	Muthuraman et al. 2011
	Saponin rich extract of *Acorus calamus* improved injury-induced neuropathic pain by virtue of its anti-oxidative, anti-inflammatory, calcium homeostasis and anti-TNF-a associated neuroprotective actions. (Nb. TNF = tumour necrosis factor).	Muthuraman and Singh, 2012
Aleurites moluc-cana L.	Constituents of *Aleurites moluccana*, mainly 2″-O-rhamnosylswertisin, revealed an anti-nociceptive effect by interacting with: – Opioid system, enhancing the descendent-control of pain; – Dopaminergic and oxidonitrergic system, reducing the central sensitization resulting from glutamate activity, and – Inflammatory components such as neutrophil migration and cytokine release (IL-1β).	Quintão et al. 2012
Aloe saponaria Haw	The topical application of *Aloe saponaria* cream (10%) diminished nociceptive behaviours from day 1 to 6 (peak at day 2). Consequently, *Aloe saponaria* revealed antinociceptive and anti-inflammatory properties in rats subjected to a thermal injury, validating its traditional use for burn injuries.	Silva et al. 2013
Cannabis sativa L.	Trans-caryophyllene, an active constituent of the plant showed marked oral antinociceptive properties in both acute and chronic models of nociception in mice. It is postulated that it may involve interaction with the opioid and endocannabinoid pathways, besides reduction of IL-1beta at the injury site.	Paula-Freire et al. 2013
	The analgesia obtained from a low dose of delta-9-tetrahydrocannabinol (1.29%) in patients, most of whom were experiencing neuropathic pain despite conventional treatments, is a clinically significant outcome.	Wilsey et al. 2013
Crocus sativus L.	A 7-day treatment with the ethanolic and aqueous extracts (50,100 and 200 mg/kg, i.p.) and its constituent, safranal (0.025, 0.05 and 0.1 mg/kg, i.p.), alleviated the behavioural symptoms of neuropathic pain in a dose - dependent manner.	Amin and Hosseinzadeh, 2012

Medicinal plants	Endorsing *in vivo* studies	References
Euphorbia tirucalli L.	The plant-derived triterpene alcohol euphol demonstrated promising anti-inflammatory and anti-nociceptive properties when dosed orally and assessed in several models of pain in mice. The suggested mode of action was due to its ability to inhibit the activation and/or release of various inflammatory mediators, among others.	Dutra et al. 2012
Gelsemium sempervirens Ait.	Gelsemine, extracted from this plant, produces potent and specific anti-nociception in chronic pain states without induction of apparent tolerance. Also, gelsemine produces anti-nociception by activation of spinal α3 glycine receptors, supporting the notion that spinal α3 glycine receptors are a potential therapeutic target molecule for management of chronic pain.	Zhang et al. 2013
St. John's Wort	SJW, acutely administered at low doses (30–60 mg kg 1 p.o.), reversed mechanical hyperalgesia with a prolonged effect in rat models, being effective up to 180 min after injection. Hyperforin and hypericin were responsible for the antihyperalgesic properties. The mode of action included phosphorylation of Protein Kinase C (PKC) and its isoforms.	Galeotti et al. 2010

Massage Therapy

Massage involves manipulation of soft tissues, using the hands or a mechanical device, and has its roots from many parts of the globe including Babylonia (around 900 BC), China (around 2700 BC), India (around 1500-120 BC), and Greece (Hippocrates 460-377 BC). Massage entails the interplay of techniques including Cyriax (a deep friction massage technique, as reviewed by Chamberlain, 1982), effleurage, petrissage, friction, kneading, or hacking and is considered one of the earliest and most pristine methods of relieving pain (Imamura et al. 2008). An analgesic effect of massage is proposed in Gate Control Theory, which postulates that pressure applied during massage travels along nerve pathways faster than pain, thereby blocking pain transmission. Consequently, massage stimulates parasympathetic feedback and inhibits sympathetic tone, thus leading the body to a relaxation mode (Wang et al. 2010).

There is mounting evidence endorsing the effectiveness of massage therapy in relieving painful conditions, including chronic low back pain (Imamura et al. 2008), pain in temporomandibular joint syndrome, characterized by chronic or acute musculoskeletal or myofascial pain

(Eisensmith, 2007), pain in patients recovering from cardiac surgery (Bauer et al. 2010; Wang et al. 2010) and metastatic bone pain (Jane et al. 2011). Recent publications emphasise that symptoms of back pain may be effectively relieved using aromatic ginger oil with Swedish massage (Sritoomma et al. 2013) and therapeutic massage (Brosseau et al. 2012).

Spinal Manipulation

Spinal manipulation is a technique that encompasses the use of force applied to specific body tissues, usually vertebral joints, to serve a therapeutic purpose. The load delivery changes with respect to velocity, amplitude, frequency, choice of lever, and direction of force application (Goertz et al. 2012). Consequently, findings from a study (Dagenais et al. 2010) demonstrate that spinal manipulation is promising in alleviating pain, in the short, intermediate, and long term. Moreover, 12 sessions of spinal manipulation in 6 weeks from a chiropractor, carried out on patients with chronic nonspecific low back pain, produced diminished pain and improved functional ability (Haas et al. 2013).

Tai Chi

Tai Chi or Tai Chi Chuan, practised since antiquity, has its roots in traditional Chinese medicine. It encompasses mild, controlled, sequential movements combined with deep diaphragmatic breathing. Tai Chi contributes to "internal harmony" by strengthening and stretching muscles and ligaments. Tai Chi exercise may be helpful in rheumatological conditions since it has beneficial effects on muscle strength, stress reduction, and bone health (Uhlig, 2012). Some studies (Lauche et al. 2013; Tsai et al. 2013) have provided evidence that Tai Chi is effective in relieving pain, improving stiffness and physical function in knee osteoarthritis patients.

Yoga

Yoga, with origins from Ayurveda, encompasses physical postures (*asana*), breathing techniques (*pranayama*), and meditation (*dyana*). Yoga is believed to enhance physical and mental well-being, by uniting mind, body, and spirit (Posadzkia et al. 2011; Cramer et al. 2013). The mechanisms by which yoga is claimed to relieve chronic and acute pain involve improvement of tissue flexibility, together with relaxation effects, and release of encephalin or endorphins. Other possible mechanisms of action are diminished sympathetic nervous system activity and reduction of pro-inflammatory mediators (Posadzkia et al. 2011).

In consequence, yoga has been demonstrated to ameliorate a cluster of physical health conditions, such as low back pain, fibromyalgia, arthritis, or irritable bowel syndrome (Cramer et al. 2013). Moreover, yoga practiced for 30 minutes at least three times per week for 10 weeks, could aid in diminishing discomfort during childbirth, reducing pain during labour and within 2 hours following delivery, and curbing the labour period (Chuntharapat et al. 2008). Another study (Michalsen et al. 2012) provided evidence of yoga as a potential alternative for effective and safe treatment of chronic neck pain.

Other CAM Therapies

Other CAM therapies for pain include aromatherapy and nutritional supplementation.

Aromatherapy is postulated to improve parasympathetic responses through effects on touch and smell, encouraging relaxation at a deep level. Some evidence demonstrates that it is useful as a complementary approach to pain management, because relaxation reportedly changes subjective perceptions of pain (Buckle, 1999).

Numerous dietary supplements, including glucosamine, bromelain, vitamins B1, B6, B12, C, zinc, and manganese, have been reported effective in management of musculoskeletal conditions including chronic low back pain. Additionally, it has been suggested that several B vitamins possess anti-nociceptive and anti-inflammatory properties (Gagnier, 2008).

Select Alternative Remedies, for Pain Management on Mauritius

The following is a summary of a study we conducted on the island, highlighting commonly used alternative therapies including herbal remedies,

Ayurvedic medicine, massage and yoga, reported to be influential in pain management and/or treatment (Sreekeesoon and Mahomoodally, 2014).

Herbal Remedies

Herbal remedies were common in the management of pain-related conditions. A total of 78 plant species distributed within 40 families, and 20 polyherbal preparations, were identified using a survey. Of particular interest, 6 indigenous/endemic plants were reported for the first time in use for pain management and/or treatment. The most significant biological plant family was Xanthorrhoeaceae. *P*lant species known to be useful in traditional medicine accounted for 11.4% of the total flora in Mauritius. *Coix lacrymajobi* (Job's Tears) was utilized as treatment for lower back ache, and *Morinda citrifolia (Morinda, or 'Noni') was frequently used for its* anti-nociceptive properties.

Ayurvedic Products

As depicted in Table 5, below, Ayurvedic products commonly used by patients, available in private Ayurvedic outlets and pharmacies, included local preparations (64.7%) used to manage numerous pain conditions. The majority of Ayurvedic preparations were polyherbal mixtures comprising of at least 10 medicinal plants. Some contained up to 30 extracts of plants and, most of the time, the composition remained undisclosed to patients. However, practitioners stated that commonly used medicinal herbs in Ayurvedic medicine included Castor-Oil plant (*Ricinus communis*), common Ginger (*Zingiber officinale*), Withania (*Withania somnifera*), Fennel (*Foeniculum vulgare*), Indian Long Pepper (*Piper longum*), Sweet Flag (*Acorus calamus*), Celery (*Apium graveolens*) and Turmeric (*Curcuma longa*).

The Ayurvedic products were readily available and imported from India. However, in the case of powders, Ayurvedic practitioners often blended 3-4 powders together, resulting in a concoction which was claimed to provide faster pain relief.

Practitioners stated that treatment duration varies from months to years. They treated patients who were extremely dissatisfied with conventional therapies, having found no pain relief at all. For pain diagnoses, they asked questions relating to pain intensity and possible causes, not restricted to physical causes. In addition, they inquired about conventional therapies the patient has used or is using, and provided counselling on which conventional drugs to avoid with Ayurvedic therapy. 65% of patients reported being satisfied with Ayurvedic therapy, although some were discouraged by the duration of treatment, which could require years, and others reported no pain relief despite a full year of therapy.

Table 5. Ayurvedic products for pain, reported by CAM users and Ayurvedic practitioners

Ayurvedic Product	Pain conditions used	Dosage form	Dosage, Mode of administration	Frequency of use (%)
Shirshuladi Vajra Ras®	Headache, migraine, feeling of heaviness in head, feeling pain in head	Powder, Capsules	1 tablet (250 mg) morning and night.	8 (5.4)
Prasarini Tail®	Inability to walk, Sciatica, Head, Neck and back stiffness	Oil	Local application 3 to 4 times daily.	5 (3.4)
Saindhavadi Tail®	Back Pain, hip joint, knee joint, chest pain, painful urination, kidney stones	Oil	Local application 3 to 4 times daily.	5 (3.4)
Sure Relief – Pain Oil®	Muscular pains, arthritis problems, back pain, joint pains and strains	Oil	Local application 3 to 4 times daily.	12 (8.1)
Amrutanajan®	Relieves pain associated with muscle injury, joint sprain, minor rheumatic pain	Joint-Muscle spray	Local application.	6 (4.0)
Shallaki® capsule	Joint care and pain release	Capsule	1-2 Capsules daily after meals.	8 (5.4)
Hamdard Balm®	Headache, sprains, Muscular pain	Balm	Local application 3 to 4 times daily.	5 (3.4)
Navratna® Oil	Headaches, migraine, body aches, joint pain, sprains and myalgias	Oil	Local application 3 to 4 times daily.	25 (16.8)
Fleximur® Oil	Inflammatory conditions including pain from arthritis	Oil	Local application 3 to 4 times daily.	4 (2.7)
Emani® Mentho Plus Balm	Backaches, musculoskeletal pains, neck stiffness, sciatica	Balm	Local application 3 to 4 times daily.	11 (7.4)

Table 5. (Continued)

Ayurvedic Product	Pain conditions used	Dosage form	Dosage, Mode of administration	Frequency of use (%)
Maha Narayan Taila®	Rheumatic pain, abdominal pain, "shooting" pain, pain in joints/muscles	Oil	Local application 3 to 4 times daily.	18 (12.1)
Maharasnadi kadha®	Sciatica, paralysis, knee/ankle joint pain	Syrup	1-2 tablespoons with equal qty of water.	4 (2.7)
Swarna Guggulu®	Joint pain, paralysis, sciatica	Capsule	1-2 capsules morning and evening.	4 (2.7)
Yograj Guggulu®	Chronic pain, rheumatic pain, umbilical pain	Capsule	1-2 capsules morning and evening.	5 (3.4)
Sinhanad Guggulu®	Joint pain	Capsule	1-2 capsules morning and evening.	6 (4.0)
Painmukti® Cream	Muscular and joint pain, stiffness, and headache	Cream	Local application 3 to 4 times daily.	4 (2.7)
Cure on® Oil	Body aches, backache, muscle pain, leg cramps, joint pain	Oil	Local application 3 to 4 times daily.	5 (3.4)
Zandu® balm	Backaches, musculoskeletal pains, neck stiffness, sciatica	Balm	Local application 3 to 4 times daily	14 (9.4)

Massage Therapy

Massage was the third most sought therapy for pain management and/or treatment. Massage therapists used techniques including cupping, Cyriax manipulation therapy, effleurage, petriss-age, friction, kneading, hacking, acupressure and stretching. The therapist could choose to work with thumbs and hands or elbows, to enable sufficient force to reach deeper muscles. A patient required 4 to 8 sessions of massage for chronic pain. Therapists also made use of aromatherapy (essential oils) during massage sessions, reporting that patients require consecutive sessions to secure maximum benefit. As depicted in Table 6, commonly used essential oils were Eucalyptus oil and Ylang Ylang oil, which survey respondents claimed aid enormously in pain relief.

Table 6. Essential oils used during massage therapy for pain management and/or treatment

Botanical name	Trade name of essential oils	Type of massages used
Cananga odorata (Lam.) Hook. f. and Thomson	Ylang Ylang	Body massage
Eucalyptus globulus Labill.	Eucalyptus	Body massage
Lavandula officinalis Chaix	Lavender	Body massage
Mentha arvensis L.	Menthol/Peppermint	Body massage
Prunus dulcis (Mill.) D.A.Webb	Almond	Head massage

Yoga

Yoga therapy was popular among CAM users in our study for pain management and/or treatment (Sreekeesoon and Mahomoodally, 2014). The majority of yoga users practised yoga exercises on a weekly basis whilst some practised the exercises on a daily basis. Most yoga users were part of yoga classes that took place in social community centres on a weekly basis. A yoga session consisted of a sequence of asanas and prayanama including specific postures that aid in pain relief. The yoga therapists placed emphasis on the fact that specific postures can be helpful in pain relief. However, because yoga therapy deals with general mind-body well-being, it is important to practice overall body postures to obtain maximum benefit. The *Surya Namaskar* (set of 12 asanas) was found be frequently used by CAM users who performed at least 3 cycles thrice or more frequently in a week. Many yoga postures were reportedly used by informants. Relaxation techniques, such as *Shavasana*, were also practiced, and contributed to the overall benefit of yoga practice. Some of the most common and specific postures that aided in pain relief are described in Table 7.

Challenges of CAM

Although users may regard CAM as “natural” and therefore safe, it may cause adverse events. Adverse events for oral herbal analgesics consist mainly of temporary gastrointestinal symptoms. For instance, Cayenne (*Capsicum annum*) when taken orally, has caused abdominal fullness, gas, bloating and nausea. *Harpagophytum procumbens* (Devil's Claw) is believed to increase secretion of stomach acid, decrease blood glucose levels and blood pressure, and possibly to interfere with cytochrome P450 (Gagnier, 2008). Moreover, exceeding doses of vitamin C (greater than 3,000 mg) may increase the half-life of acetaminophen from 2.3 to 3.1 hours (Gagnier, 2008).

Table 7. Yoga asanas (postures) and pranayama (breathing exercises) used for pain management and/or treatment as reported by CAM users and yoga therapists

Yoga (postures and breathing techniques)		Indications	Frequency (%)
Sanskrit name	English name		
Surya Namaskar	Sun salutation	A set with 12 steps, used for general body wellbeing; aids in backaches, sciatica, pain in spinal area.	25 (23.8)
Anantasana	God Vishnu's Resting pose	Sciatica	5 (4.8)
Setu Bandha Sarvaṅgasana	Bridge pose	Back aches	8 (7.6)
Halasana	Plough pose	Stiffness of back and shoulders	4 (3.8)
Bhujangasana	Cobra pose	High and mid-back aches, slipped discs and sciatica	6 (5.7)
Salabhasana	Locust pose	Upper, mid and low back aches	7 (6.7)
Matsyasana	Fish pose	Stiffness of shoulder and ankle joints	5 (4.8)
Dhanurasana	Bow pose	Back aches and mild disc problems	6 (5.7)
Urdhva Dhanurasana	Upward bow pose	Back aches, early disc problems and sciatica	4 (3.8)
Pascimottananasana	Back Spine Stretching pose	Back aches and arthritis	5 (4.8)
Kapalbhathi	Breathing exercise		20 (19.0)
Agnisa	Breathing exercise		10 (9.5)

Other challenges to CAM use include the complexity of CAM modalities, possible interactions between CAM and conventional therapies, lack of professional satisfaction among CAM therapists and the prolonged duration of certain CAM treatments. Therapists have coined the phrase "healing crisis" to describe how symptoms of illnesses treated with CAM are in some aggravated before they improve. With concerns increasing around issues of safety in health care, individual professional CAM practitioners have a responsibility to ensure safety of their products and practices, as much as possible. Global partnerships between experts in the field, including practitioners and researchers, could help achieve required levels of expertise (White et al., 2013).

CONCLUSION

Chronic pain unequivocally remains challenging to assess and treat, with negative repercussions on the daily life of individuals. Common chronic pain conditions including sciatica, rheumatoid arthritis and fibromyalgia have been briefly reviewed in this chapter. Conventional therapies such as analgesics and NSAIDs, despite their effectiveness, remain inadequate in managing and treating mild and chronic pain-related conditions. Owing to potential cumulative toxicity and side-effects, as distinct constraints of mainstream medicine, and with a renaissance of alternative medicine in current years, panoply of commonly used alternative therapies, with their reported effectiveness in relation to pain management has also been reviewed.

A remarkable number of plant species offer potential analgesic and/or anti-nociceptive properties. Information about their potential in pain therapy is recapitulated in this chapter, which serves to emphasise the need to undertake further ethnopharmacological investigations that would discern new therapeutic options for pain management using traditional herbal medicine.

REFERENCES

Adachi, N., Munesada, M., Yamada, N., Suzuki, H., Futohashi, A., Shigeeda, T., Kato, S., and Nishigaki, M., 2013. Effects of Aromatherapy Massage on Face-Down Posture-Related Pain After Vitrectomy: A Randomized Controlled Trial. *Pain Management Nursing*, 2013, doi: 10.1016/j.pmn.2012.12.004.

Agunu, A., Dafam, G. D., and Kagaru, D. C., 2009. Medicinal plants used in traditional pain management in Jos, Nigeria. *Planta Medica*, 75 - PJ202.

Aickin, M., Mccaffery, A., Pugh, G., Tick, H., Ritenbaugh, C., Hicks, P., Pelletier, K.R., Cao, J., Himick, D., and Monahan, J., 2013. Description of a clinical stream of back-pain patients based on electronic medical records. *Complementary Therapies in Clinical Practice*, 19 (3): 158-176.

Alfaro, N., Lázaro, P., Gabriele, G., Garcia-Vicuña, R., Jover, J.A., And Sevilla, J., 2013. Perceptions, Attitudes and Experiences of Family Caregivers of Patients with Musculoskeletal Diseases: A Qualitative Approach. *Reumatología Clínica*, 9 (6): 334-339.

Allen, K. D., and Nelson, A. E., 2013. Chapter 96–Osteoarthritis and Other Musculoskeletal Diseases. Women and Health (Second Edition) Pages 1415–1429.

Amin, B., and Hosseinzadeh, H., 2012. Evaluation of aqueous and ethanolic extracts of saffron, *Crocus sativus* L., and its constituents, safranal and crocin in allodynia and hyperalgesia induced by chronic constriction injury model of neuropathic pain in rats. *Fitoterapia,* 83 (5): 888–895.

Arendt, K.W., and Tessmer-Tuck, J.A., 2013. Nonpharmacologic Labor Analgesia. *Clinics in Perinatology*, 40 (3): 351–371.

Arome, D., Sunday, A. I., Onalike, E.I., And Amarachi, A., 2014. Pain and inflammation: Management by conventional and herbal therapy. *Indian Journal of Pain*, 28: 1.

Bashir, U., and Colvin, L.A., 2012. The place of pharmacological treatment in chronic pain. *Anaesthesia and intensive care medicine*, 14: 12.

Bauer, B.A., Cutshall, S. M., Wentworth, L. J., Engen, D., Messner, K. P., Wood, C. M., Brekke, K. M., Kelly, R. F., and Sundt, T. M., 2010. Effect of massage therapy on pain, anxiety, and tension after cardiac surgery: A randomized study. *Complementary Therapies in Clinical Practice*, 16 (2): 70–75.

Berman, R. L. H., Iris, M.A., Bode, R., and Drengenberg, C., 2009. The Effectiveness of an Online Mind-Body Intervention for Older Adults With Chronic Pain. *The Journal of Pain*, 10 (1): 68-79.

Brosseau, L., Wells, G.A., Poitras, S., Tugwell, P., Casimiro, L., Novikov, M., Loew, L., Sredic, D., Clément, S., Gravelle, A., Kresic, D., Hua, K., Lakic, A., Ménard, G., Sabourin, S., Bolduc, M.A., Ratté, I., Mcewan, J., Furlan, A.D., Gross, A., Dagenais, S., Dryden, T., Muckenheim, R., Côté, R., Paré, V., Rouhani, A., Léonard, G., Finestone, H.M., Laferrière, L., Haines-Wangda, A., Russell-Doreleyers, M., De Angelis, G., And Cohoon. C., 2012. Ottawa Panel evidence-based clinical practice guidelines on therapeutic massage for low back pain. *Journal of Bodywork and Movement Therapies*, 16 (4): 424e455.

Bruckenthal, P., 2010. Integrating Nonpharmacologic and Alternative Strategies Into a Comprehensive Management Approach for Older Adults With Pain. *Pain Management Nursing*, 11 (2): S23-S31.

Buckle, J., 1999. Use of aromatherapy as a complementary treatment for chronic pain. *Alternative therapies in Health and Medicine*, 5 (5): 42-51.

Chamberlain, G.J., 1982. Cyriax's Friction Massage: A Review. *The journal of orthopaedic and sports physical therapy*.

Chuntharapat, S., Petpichetchian, W., and Hatthakit U., 2008. Yoga during pregnancy: Effects on maternal comfort, labor pain and birth outcomes. *Complementary Therapies in Clinical Practice*, 14 (2): 105-115.

Cramer, H., Lauche, R., Langhorst, J., Paul, A., Michalsen, A., and Dobos, G., 2013. Predictors of yoga use among internal medicine patients. *BMC Complementary and Alternative Medicine* 2013, 13: 172.

Da Silva, K.A., Manjavachi, M.N., Paszcuk, A.F., Pivatto, M., Viegas, C., Jr., Bolzani, V.S., and Calixto, J.B., 2012. Plant derived alkaloid (-)-cassine induces anti-inflammatory and anti-hyperalgesics effects in both acute and chronic inflammatory and neuropathic pain models. *Neuropharmacology*, 62 (2): 967-977.

Dagenais, S., Gay, R.E., Tricco, A.C., Freeman, M.D., And Mayer, J.M., 2010. NASS Contemporary Concepts in Spine Care: Spinal manipulation therapy for acute low back pain. *The Spine Journal*, 10 (10): 918–940.

Dailey, D. L., Rakel, B. A., Vance, C. G. T., Liebano, R. E., Amrit, A.S., Bush, H.M., Lee, K. S., Lee, J. E. and Sluka, K. A., 2013. Transcutaneous electrical nerve stimulation reduces pain, fatigue and hyperalgesia while restoring central inhibition in primary fibromyalgia. *PAIN*, 154 (11): 2554-2562.

Dorsher, P.T., 2011. Acupuncture for chronic pain. *Techniques in Regional Anesthesia and Pain Management*, 15 (2): 55–63.

Driessen, B., 2007. Pain: From Sign to Disease. *Clinical Techniques in Equine Practice*, 6: 120-125.

Dutra, R.C., Simão Da Silva, K.A., Bento, A.F., Marcon, R., Paszcuk, A.F., Meotti, F.C., Pianowski, L.F., And Calixto, J.B., 2012. Euphol, a tetracyclic triterpene produces antinociceptive effects in inflammatory and neuropathic pain: The involvement of cannabinoid system. *Neuropharmacology*, 63 (4): 593e605.

Edwards, R.R., Klick, B., Buenaver, L., Max, M.B., Haythornthwaite, J.A., Keller, R.B., and Atlas, S.J., 2007. Symptoms of distress as prospective predictors of pain-related sciatica treatment outcomes. *Pain*, 130 (1-2): 47-55.

Eisensmith, L.P., 2007. Massage therapy decreases frequency and intensity of symptoms related to temporomandibular joint syndrome in one case study. *Journal of Bodywork and Movement Therapies*, 11: 223-230.

El Barzouhi, A., Vleggeert-Lankamp, C.L., Van Der Kallen, B.F., Lycklama À Nijeholt, G.J., Van Den Hout, W.B., Koes, B.W., Peul, W.C., 2014. Back pain's association with vertebral end-plate signal changes in sciatica. *The Spine Journal*, 14 (2): 225-233.

Fouladbakhsh, J.M., Szczesny, S., Jenuwine, E.S., And Vallerand, A.H., 2011. Nondrug Therapies for Pain Management Among Rural Older Adults. *Pain Management Nursing*, 12 (2): 70-81.

GAGNIER, J.J., 2008. Evidence-informed management of chronic low back pain with herbal, vitamin, mineral, and homeopathic supplements. *The Spine Journal*, 8, 70-79.

Galeotti, N., Vivoli, E., Bilia, A.R., Vincieri, F.F., And Ghelardini, C., 2010. St. John's Wort reduces neuropathic pain through a hypericin-mediated inhibition of the protein kinase C gamma and epsilon activity. *Biochemical Pharmacology*, 79 (9): 1327–1336.

Gantenbein, A.R., Afra, J., Jenni, W., And Sândor, P.S., 2012. Complementary and alternative treatments for migraine. *Techniques in regional anesthesia and pain management*, 16 (1): 76-81.

Goertz, C.M., Pohlman, K.A., Vining, R.D., Brantingham, J.W., and Long, C.R., 2012. Patient-centered outcomes of high-velocity, low-amplitude spinal manipulation for low back pain: A systematic review. *Journal of Electromyography and Kinesiology*, 22 (5): 670-691.

Grillo, C.M., Wada, R.S., and De Sousa, M. Da L.R., 2013. Acupuncture in the Management of Acute Dental Pain. *Journal of Acupuncture and Meridian Studies*, 2013. doi: http://dx.doi.org/10.1016/j.jams.2013.03.005.

Gutiérrez, R.M., Mitchell, S., And Solis, R.V., 2008. Psidium guajava: a review of its traditional uses, phytochemistry and pharmacology. *Journal of Ethnopharmacology*, 117 (1): 1–27.

Haas, M., Vavrek, D., Peterson, D., Polissar, N., and Neradilek, M.B., 2013. Dose-response and efficacy of spinal manipulation for care of chronic low back pain: a randomized controlled trial. *The Spine Journal*, 2013.

Huguet, A., Stinson, J. N., and Mcgrath, P. J., 2010. Measurement of self-reported pain intensity in children and adolescents. *Journal of Psychosomatic Research*, 68: 329–336.

IASP Taxonomy, 2012. Available from: http://www.iasp-pain.org/AM/Template.cfm?Section=Pain_Definitions [Accessed 21 September 2013].

Imamura, M., Furlan, A.D., Dryden, T., And Irvin, E., 2008. Evidence-informed management of chronic low back pain with massage. *The Spine Journal*, 8 (1): 121-133.

Jane, S.W., Chen, S.L., Wilkie, D.J., Lin, Y.C., Foreman, S.W., Beaton, R.D., Fan, J.Y., Lu, M.Y., Wang, Y.Y., Lin, Y.H., and Liao, M.N., 2011. Effects of massage on pain, mood status, relaxation, and sleep in Taiwanese patients with metastatic bone pain: A randomized clinical trial. *PAIN*, 152 (10): 2432-2442.

Juárez-Vázquez, M.Del C., Carranza-Álvarez, C., Alonso-Castro, A.J., González-Alcaraz, V.F., Bravo-Acevedo, E., Chamarro-Tinajero, F.J., Solano, E., 2013. Ethnobotany of medicinal plants used in Xalpatlahuac, Guerrero, México. Journal of Ethnopharmacology, 148 (2): 521-527.

Kirby, E.R., Brooma, A.F., Sibbritt, D.W., Adams, J., and Refshauge, K.M., 2013. A national cross-sectional survey of back pain care amongst Australian women aged 60-65. *European Journal of Integrative Medicine*, 5: 36-43.

Lacroix, D., Prado, S., Kamoga, D., Kasenene, J., Namukobe, J., Krief, S., Dumontet, V., Mouray, E., Bodo, B., and Brunois, F., 2011. Antiplasmodial and cytotoxic activities of medicinal plants traditionally used in the village of Kiohima, Uganda. *Journal of Ethnopharmacology*, 133 (2): 850-855.

Lauche, R., Langhorst, J., Dobos, G., and Cramer, H., 2013. A systematic review and meta-analysis of Tai Chi for osteoarthritis of the knee. *Complementary Therapies in Medicine*, 21 (4): 396-406.

Lee, S., Kim, K. H., Kim, T. H., Kim, J. E., Kim, J. H., Kang, J. W., Kang, K. W., Jung, S. Y., Kim, A. R., Park, H.J., Shin, M.S., Hong, K. E., Song, H. S., Choi, J.B., Kim, H.J., and Choi, S. M., 2013. Moxibustion for treating knee osteoarthritis: study protocol of a multicentre randomized controlled trial. *BMC Complementary and Alternative Medicine*, 13: 59.

Lewandowski, W., and Jacobson, A., 2013. Bridging the Gap Between Mind and Body: A Biobehavioral Model of the Effects of Guided Imagery on Pain, Pain Disability, and Depression. Pain Management Nursing, 14 (4): 368-378.

Majumdar, S., Wendy Thompson, W., Naveed Ahmad, N., Catherine Gordon, C., And Addison, C., 2013. The use and effectiveness of complementary and alternative medicine for pain in sickle cell anemia. *Complementary Therapies in Clinical Practice*, 1e4.

Michalsen, A., Traitteur, H., Lüdtke, R., Brunnhuber, S., Meier, L., Jeitler, M., Büssing, A., and Kessler, C., 2012. Yoga for Chronic Neck Pain: A Pilot

Randomized Controlled Clinical Trial. *The Journal of Pain*, 13 (11): 1122-1130.

Mosaddegh, M., Naghibi, F., Moazzeni, H., Pirani, A., And Esmaeili, S., 2012. Ethnobotanical survey of herbal remedies traditionally used in Kohghiluyeh va Boyer Ahmad province of Iran. *Journal of Ethnopharmacology*, 141 (1): 80-95.

Murthy, V., Sibbritt, D., Adams, J., Broom, A., Kirby, E., And Refshauge, K.M., 2014. Self-prescribed complementary and alternative medicine use for back pain amongst a range of care options: Results from a nationally representative sample of 1,310 women aged 60-65 years. *Complementary Therapies in Medicine*, 22 (1): 133-40.

Muthuraman, A., And Singh, N., 2012. Neuroprotective effect of saponin rich extract of *Acorus calamus* L. in rat model of chronic constriction injury (CCI) of sciatic nerve-induced neuropathic pain. *Journal of Ethnopharmacology*, 142 (3): 723-731.

Muthuraman, A., Singh, N., and Jaggi, A.S., 2011. Protective effect of Acorus calamus L. in rat model of vincristine induced painful neuropathy: An evidence of anti-inflammatory and anti-oxidative activity. *Food and Chemical Toxicology* 49 (10): 2557-2563.

National Centre for Complementary and Alternative Medicine. Chronic Pain and CAM: At a Glance. NCCAM, 2011.

Available from: http://nccam.nih.gov/health/pain/chronic.htm [Accessed 30 September 2013].

National Centre for Complementary and Alternative Medicine. What is Complementary and Alternative Medicine? NCCAM, 2012. Available at: http://nccam.nih.gov/sites/nccam.nih.gov/files/D347_05-25-2012.pdf [Accessed 30 November 2013].

Paiva, S., and Carneiro, M. M., 2013. Complementary and Alternative Medicine in the Treatment of Chronic Pelvic Pain in Women: What Is the Evidence? *ISRN Pain*, 2013.

Paula-Freire, L. I., Andersen, M. L., Gama, V. S., Molska, G. R., and Carlini, E. L., 2013. The oral administration of trans-caryophyllene attenuates acute and chronic pain in mice. *Phytomedicine*, 2013.

Peacock, J., 2013. TENS and acupuncture therapy for soft tissue pain. *Anaesthesia and Intensive Care Medicine*, 14 (11): 502-504.

Peleg, R., Liberman, O., Press, Y., and Shvartzman, P., 2011. Patients visiting the complementary medicine clinic for pain: a cross sectional study. *BMC Complementary and Alternative Medicine*, 11: 36.

Plastaras, C. T., Schran, S., Kim, N., Sorosky, S., Darr, D., Chen, M.S., And Lansky, R., 2011. Complementary and Alternative Treatment for Neck Pain: Chiropractic, Acupuncture, TENS, Massage, Yoga, Tai Chi, and Feldenkrais. *Physical Medicine and Rehabilitation Clinics of North America*, 22 (3): 521-537.

Poole, H., Glenn, S., And Murphy, P., 2007. A randomised controlled study of reflexology for the management of chronic low back pain. *European Journal of Pain*, 11 (8): 878-887.

Posadzki, P., Lewandowski, W., Terry, R., Ernst, E., And Stearns, A., 2012. Guided Imagery for Non-Musculoskeletal Pain: A Systematic Review of Randomized Clinical Trials. *Journal of Pain and Symptom Management*, 44: 1.

Posadzkia, P., Ernsta, E., Terrya, R., and Leea, M.S., 2011. Is yoga effective for pain? A systematic review of randomized clinical trials. *Complementary Therapies in Medicine*, 19: 281-287.

Powell, R.A., Downing, J., Ddungu, H., And Mwangi-Powell, F.N., 2010. Chapter 10-Pain History and Pain Assessment. *Guide to Pain Management in Low-Resource Settings*, 2010.

Quintão, N. L., Antonialli, C. S., Da Silva, G. F., Rocha, L. W., De Souza, M. M., Malheiros, A., Meyre-Silva, C., Lucinda-Silva, R. M., Bresolin, T. M., And Filho, V.C., 2012. *Aleurites moluccana* and its main active ingredient, the flavonoid 2″-O-rhamnosylswertisin, have promising antinociceptive effects in experimental models of hypersensitivity in mice. *Pharmacology, Biochemistry and Behavior*, 102 (2): 302-311.

Rehberg, B., 2010. Evidence-based integrative pain medicine. *European Journal of Integrative Medicine*, 2: 109-113.

Ren, X. M., Cao, J. J., Shen, X. Y., Wang, L. Z., Zhao, L., Wu, F., and Zhang, H.M., 2012. Preliminary clinical randomized controlled trial on knee osteoarthritis treated with moxibustion. *World Journal of acupuncture – Moxibustion*, 22 (2): 28-33.

Schofield, P., 2012. Pain management in older adults. *MEDICINE*, 41: 1.

Silva, M. A., Trevisan, G., Klafke, J. Z., Rossato, M. F., Walker, C. I., Oliveira, S. M., Silva, C. R., Boligon, A. A., Flores, F. C., De Bona Silva, C., Athayde, M. L., And Ferreira, J., 2013. Antinociceptive and anti-inflammatory effects of *Aloe saponaria* Haw on thermal injury in rats. *Journal of Ethnopharmacology*, 146 (1): 393-401.

Sreekeesoon, D. P., and Mahomoodally, M. F., 2014. Ethnopharmacological analysis of medicinal plants and animals used in the treatment and management of pain in Mauritius. *Journal of Ethnopharmacology*, 157: 181-200.

Sritoomma, N., Moyle, W., Cooke, M., and O'dwyer, S., 2013. The effectiveness of Swedish massage with aromatic ginger oil in treating chronic low back pain in older adults: A randomized controlled trial. *Complementary Therapies in Medicine*, 2013.

Steeds, C. E., 2009. The anatomy and physiology of pain. *Surgery*, 27: 12.

Terhorst, L., Schneider, M. J., Kim, K. H., Goozdich, L. M., and Stilley, C. S., 2011. Complementary and alternative medicine in the treatment of pain in fibromyalgia: a systematic review of randomized controlled trials. *Journal of Manipulative and Physiological Therapeutics*, 2011.

Tournaire, M., and Theau-Yonneau, A., 2007. Complementary and Alternative Approaches to Pain Relief During Labor. *Advance Access Publication*, 4 (4): 409-417.

Tracy, B., And Morrison, R.S., 2013. Pain Management in Older Adults. *Clinical Therapeutics*, 35: 11.

Tsai, P. F., Chang, J. Y., Beck, C., Kuo, Y. F., and Keefe, F. J., 2013. A Pilot Cluster-Randomized Trial of a 20-Week Tai Chi Program in Elders With Cognitive Impairment and Osteoarthritic Knee: Effects on Pain and Other Health Outcomes. *Journal of Pain and Symptom Management*, 45 (4): 660-669.

Turk, D.C., Wilson, H. D., and Cahana, A., 2011. Treatment of chronic non-cancer pain. *Lancet*, 377: 2226-35.

Uhlig, T., 2012. Tai Chi and yoga as complementary therapies in rheumatologic conditions. *Best Practice and Research Clinical Rheumatology*, 26: 387-398.

Verkamp, E. K., Flowers, S. R., Lynch-Jordan, A. M., Taylor, J., Ting, V. T., and Kashikar-Zuck, S., 2013. A Survey of Conventional and Complementary Therapies Used by Youth with Juvenile-Onset Fibromyalgia. *Pain Management Nursing*, 14 (4): e244-e250.

Vitalini, S., Iriti, M., Puricelli, C., Ciuchi, D., Segale, A., and Fico, G., 2013. Traditional knowledge on medicinal and food plants used in Val San Giacomo (Sondrio, Italy)--an alpine ethnobotanical study. *Journal of Ethnopharmacology*, 145 (2): 517-29.

Vitetta, L., Cicuttini, F., and Sali, A., 2008. Alternative therapies for musculoskeletal conditions. *Best Practice and Research Clinical Rheumatology*, 22 (3): 499-522.

Wambugu, S. N., Mathiu, P. M., Gakuya, D. W., Kanui, T. I., Kabasa, J. D., And Kiama, S.G., 2011. Medicinal plants used in the management of chronic joint pains in Machakos and Makueni counties, Kenya. Journal of Ethnopharmacology, 137 (2): 945-955.

Wang, A. T., Sundt, T. M., Cutshall, S. M., and Bauer, B. A., 2010. Massage Therapy After Cardiac Surgery. *Semin Thoracic Surg*, 22 (3): 225-229.

WHO guidelines on the pharmacological treatment of persisting pain in children with medical illnesses. WHO, 2012. Available from:http://www.who.int/medicines/areas/quality_safety/guide_perspainchild/en/ [Accessed 14 October 2013].

Wilsey, B., Marcotte, T., Deutsch, R., Gouaux, B., Sakai, S., And Donaghe, H., 2013. Low-Dose Vaporized Cannabis Significantly Improves Neuropathic Pain. *The Journal of Pain*, 14 (2): 136-148.

Wirth, J. H., Hudgins, J.C., and Paice, J. A., 2005. Use of Herbal Therapies to Relieve Pain: A Review of Efficacy and Adverse Effects. *Pain Management Nursing*, 6 (4): 145–167.

Yoon, S. L. And Kim, J. H., 2013. Factors contributing to the use of complementary and alternative medicine in rural older women with chronic pain in South Korea. *Applied Nursing Research*, 26:186-191.

Zareba, G., 2009. Phytotherapy for pain relief. *Drugs Today (Barc)*. 45 (6): 445-67.

Zhang, J. Y., Gong, N., Huang, J. L., Guo, L. C., and Wang, Y. X., 2013. Gelsemine, a principal alkaloid from *Gelsemium sempervirens* Ait., exhibits potent and specific antinociception in chronic pain by acting at spinal α3 glycine receptors. *Pain*, 154 (11): 2452-62.

In: Alternative Medicine ISBN: 978-1-63484-826-8
Editors: E. P. Cherniack and T. Holmes © 2016 Nova Science Publishers, Inc.

Chapter 7

THE POTENTIAL FOR LAUGHTER AND HUMOR THERAPY IN THE ELDERLY

E. Paul Cherniack

Geriatrics and Extended Care Service and Geriatric Research, Education, and Clinical Center (GRECC) of the Miami Veterans Affairs Medical Center, and the Division of Geriatrics and Palliative Medicine, University of Miami Miller School of Medicine, Miami, FL, US

ABSTRACT

Laughter therapy refers to a treatment modality in which a facilitator induces or trains patients to laugh (with or without humor) to obtain physiologic or psychological benefit. Related, but not synonymous modalities include humor therapy, which specifically uses humor as a treatment to improve the health of patients which may not necessarily involve laughter, and laughter yoga, a type of exercise developed by an Indian physician in which a therapist leads patients to clap, chant stretch, breathe, and laugh without the inducement of humor [1, 2]. All of these modalities may confer related health benefits, though laughter and humor therapy have not been studied as intensively as laughter yoga.

INTRODUCTION

The anatomic basis for laughter is uncertain. Laughter regulation occurs in the dorsal upper pons with both" a voluntary" pathway extending to the ventral brain stem, and an "involuntary (emotional) pathway" projecting to the thalamus, subthalamus, hypothalamus, and amygdale [1]. There is auditory processing of laughter in the right dorsolateral inferior frontal gyrus [1]. Laughter results in heightened serum concentrations of oxytocin, which may account for its benefits [1]. Oxytocin lowers cortisol concentrations and suppresses the amygdale [1].

Induction of laughter per se causes short-term physiologic benefits which may last longer. Laughter stimulates breathing, heart rate, and augments cardiac output. Combined with exercise, laughter may decrease blood pressure [3]. Viewing humor lowers cortisol concentrations and stimulates immunocyte activity while reducing proinflammatory cytokine concentrations [3].

Interestingly, while there is much stability in the response to humorous stimuli with age, there may be changes in the ability to elicit laughter or to perceive humor with age [4]. One study suggested the elderly laugh less with age, but sense of humor, associated with satisfaction with life, maintains constancy [5].

EVIDENCE FOR LAUGHTER AS THERAPY IN THE ELDERLY

Two studies imply that laughter and humor therapy can improve quality of life in a population of elderly not selected for specific illnesses. In an open study, seventy-two retired persons, all at least age 60, in Iran participated in either bi-weekly hour and a half interventions lasting one and a half months or a control group that did not attend these sessions [6]. Investigators assessed subjects on the 28-item General Health Questionnaire. Both groups improved their scores during the intervention, but those who received the intervention scored a mean of between one and two extra points better in anxiety, insomnia, somatic symptoms and general health subscales of the General Health Questionnaire.

In a second trial, twenty-seven participants, all at least sixty years old, enrolled in weekly two-hour laughter and exercise sessions for three months [7]. Half the group attended began immediately, the other half after three months. During the sessions, subjects viewed comedy for 50 minutes, undertook seated exercise not further described, and received a 10 minute talk about pertinent health topics. Those who attended intervention sessions immediately had a significantly higher bone mineral density, HgA1c, and an improvement in self-reported health at the conclusion of their participation in the trial than those who delayed treatment sessions.

Laughter and humor therapy in preliminary trials has been used to improve cognitive and mental health. In one qualitative study, English day care patients with dementia participated in a program during which acting instructors engaged subjects in four workshops lasting two or three hours weekly to help create a "mockumentary film." Relatives who were caregivers of the subjects informed investigators in a subsequent discussion group that the subjects appeared to improve their communication skills as a result of the project [8].

Sixty other depressed individuals, ages 60-80, who attended a community center in Iran experienced ten sessions of laughter yoga, aerobic exercise, or an unspecified control intervention [9]. Both laughter yoga and aerobic exercise participants, all of whom initially scored at least 10 on the 30-point Geriatric Depression scale, noted a five point improvement. In another trial, residents from 35 different nursing homes encountered "ElderClowns," as trained therapists that conducted 9 to 12 sessions [10]. Control subjects received care without this clown therapy. Clowning sessions included telling jokes, playing music, and conversation. Nursing home staff were trained to assess the subjects across 14 domains of mood and behavior according to a 3 point rating scale. Attendees of the therapy scored significantly higher in four of the domains rated.

The utility of laughter and humor therapy in treating cognitive and mental disorders may extend from dementia to depression. Several preliminary studies have delineated the potential of such treatment. In one trial, 99 subjects whose score on the 15-point Geriatric Depression Scale was greater than four, and who either resided on inpatient wards or attended a clinic in Germany took part in four ninety-minute humor group treatments that occurred twice weekly, and included 7 to 12 patients or conventional group and individual psychotherapy and pharmacotherapy [11]. Each session focused on a specific humorous task, such as reminiscing over humorous events, examining unusual objects found in a bag, or comedic role-playing. Both intervention and control groups significantly improved their mean depression scale scores by 39 and 29 percent respectively. However, the humor groups accrued a greater self-rated score for life satisfaction on a 26 point scale, while the control group did not.

In a second trial from the same institution of 90 patients with major depression patients (GDS score at least 8), humor therapy did not reduce depressive symptoms beyond the level achieved by conventional therapy, although participants in humor therapy scored higher on a scale of life satisfaction and resilience [12]. In another investigation, 109 depressed subjects all at least age 65, experienced either four weekly 60 minute sessions in which a nurse encouraged participants to laugh, sing, and meditate or did not attend sessions [13, 14]. The mean score of participants of laughter therapy sessions was significantly lowered by one point from 7.98 to 6.94 on the Geriatric Depression Scale. This reduction did not occur in control subjects. While mean scores on the Pittsburgh Sleep Quality Index, a 0-21 scale with scores increasing with greater insomnia, deteriorated slightly in the control group, from 8.08 to 8.43, these scores improved in the intervention group from 7.98 to 6.94, $p = 0.027$.

Another trial of laughter therapy implies a role in the treatment of insomnia. In a Korean study, Investigators questioned attendees of a community center for sleep disturbance, and 109 subjects, all at least 65 years old, participated in laughter therapy or conventional care [14]. Recipients of laughter therapy improved scores on the Insomnia Severity Index and Pittsburgh Sleep Quality Index by approximately ten percent.

The benefits of laughter therapy may encompass in physical health conditions, including those with mental health implications, such as cancer. In one trial, 62 Koreans attending an outpatient radiation therapy clinic, all free of cognitive and psychiatric illness, met with a nurse trained in laughter therapy for hourly treatments on three days or received usual care [15]. The sessions involved laughing and rhythmic movements to music. Subjects rated their mood before and after the intervention using the 30 question Brief Profile of Mood States questionnaire. Participants in laughter therapy experienced significant improvements (from 1.67 to 3.55 points on a 4 point scale) for domains of depression, anger, vigor, fatigue, tension, and total mood disturbance, which was not the case for those uninvolved in the intervention sessions. Forty-one Japanese cancer patients receiving chemotherapeutic or surgical treatment engaged in laughter therapy for a minimum of 15 minutes a day that emphasized humorous role playing, and positive thinking, or received treatment without laughter therapy [16]. Those obtaining laughter therapy experienced in a significantly improved score on a scale measuring T cell functions. An additional study included 37 Koreans undergoing radiation therapy for breast cancer [17]. Patients in the group who experienced laughter therapy had lower grades of radiation-induced dermatitis than a control group lacking laughter.

Several other studies piloted a role for laughter therapy in renal failure and emphysema.

Some of these piloted the effect of laughter therapy in COPD, with mixed results thus far. In one trial, nineteen COPD patients and ten normal individuals viewed a professional clown presentation for half an hour or continued with usual therapy [18]. The subjects were videotaped, and had pulmonary function testing between 2 hours and two days after the intervention. Residual volume fell in COPD participants receiving laughter therapy, unlike controls. In another investigation, twenty-two subjects with COPD (mean age 66.9) after measurements of sense of humor, functionality and quality of life observed humorous or instructional videos for 30 minutes before receiving pulmonary function testing [19]. Investigators recorded subjects watching the videos to determine how much laughter took place. The amount of laughter correlated with worse pulmonary function.

A few additional trials suggest an effect for laughter on an intracellular level in chronic disease. In one investigation, ten diabetics had blood samples collected on two days, one of which was after watching a humorous video [20]. Exposure to humor led to lowered post-prandial blood glucose concentrations, and increased the expression of 39 genes in a microarray analysis. In another, 23 diabetics observing a comedy video experienced augmentation of serum concentrations of prorenin and heightened expression of a gene coding for a prorenin receptor gene [21]. An additional study compared cytokine levels in 41 rheumatoid arthritis patients and 23 controls in presence of a humor video [22]. Rheumatoid arthritis patients had lower interleukin-6 and higher IL-4 after laughing. In one investigation, however, 27 breast cancer patients treated with chemotherapy as subjects who engaged in laughter therapy sessions did not display altered T and B cell composition [23].

DIRECTIONS FOR FURTHER RESEARCH

In order for laughter to be able to fulfill its potential as therapy, several issues need to be addressed in further research. An important initial consideration is the use of controls in such trials. Thus far, no one has performed a blinded investigation of humor or laughter. In order to design an appropriate control condition, investigators require greater insight into the mechanism and action of the intervention. Therefore, a related issue is the discrimination between the effects of laughter and humor, which may, in fact be considerably different depending on how the therapy is applied. The effects of laughter and humor may be additive or separate in different health disorders, as was apparent on the pulmonary function of COPD patients. An important potential benefit might be that it offers a medication-free method to deliver treatment, particularly important in the elderly, in which polypharmacy is far too common.

Understanding how laughter and humor therapy affect health will foster the development of practical methods for the delivery of such therapies. Health care professionals will need to take into account other considerations in order to make appropriate use of these modalities. Patients treated with laughter or humor, might be taught by a trained instructor, at least initially, or by printed learning materials and audio-visual media. The need to employ a trained instructor, and creation and provision of certain types of media potentially add significantly to the cost of such an intervention. Elderly individuals often have sensory and cognitive impairments that pose additional challenges to learning. These and other details require clarification to determine if laughter and humor can fulfill a promise and potential of benefiting health in the elderly.

REFERENCES

[1] Woodbury-Farina MA, Antongiorgi JL. Humor. *Psychiatric Clinics of North America.* 2014;37: 561-578.

[2] Kataria M. What happens in a laughter yoga session. Available from URL: http://laughteryoga.org/english/laughteryoga/details/226 [accessed June 22. 21015.

[3] Mora-Ripoll R. The therapeutic value of laughter in medicine. *Altern Ther Health Med.* 2010;16: 56-64.

[4] Hirsch RD, Ruch W. [Cheerfulness and humor in older age: results of current studies]. *Zeitschrift fur Gerontologie und Geriatrie.* 2010;43: 5-7.

[5] Ruch W, Proyer RT, Weber M. Humor as a character strength among the elderly: theoretical considerations. *Zeitschrift fur Gerontologie und Geriatrie.* 2010;43: 8-12.

[6] Ghodsbin F, Sharif Ahmadi Z, Jahanbin I, Sharif F. The effects of laughter therapy on general health of elderly people referring to

jahandidegan community center in shiraz, iran, 2014: a randomized controlled trial. *Int J Community Based Nurs Midwifery*. 2015;3: 31-38.

[7] Hirosaki M, Ohira T, Kajiura M, et al. Effects of a laughter and exercise program on physiological and psychological health among community-dwelling elderly in Japan: randomized controlled trial. *Geriatr Gerontol Int.* 2013;13: 152-160.

[8] Hafford-Letchfield T. Funny things happen at the Grange: introducing comedy activities in day services to older people with dementia--innovative practice. *Dementia* (London). 2013;12: 840-852.

[9] Shahidi M, Mojtahed A, Modabbernia A, et al. Laughter yoga versus group exercise program in elderly depressed women: a randomized controlled trial. *Int J Geriatr Psychiatry*. 2011;26: 322-327.

[10] Low LF, Goodenough B, Fletcher J, et al. The effects of humor therapy on nursing home residents measured using observational methods: the SMILE cluster randomized trial. *J Am Med Dir Assoc*. 2014;15: 564-569.

[11] Konradt B, Hirsch RD, Jonitz MF, Junglas K. Evaluation of a standardized humor group in a clinical setting: a feasibility study for older patients with depression. *Int J Geriatr Psychiatry*. 2013;28: 850-857.

[12] Hirsch RD, Junglas K, Konradt B, Jonitz MF. [Humor therapy in the depressed elderly: results of an empirical study]. *Zeitschrift fur Gerontologie und Geriatrie*. 2010;43: 42-52.

[13] Ko HJ, Youn CH. Effects of laughter therapy on depression, cognition and sleep among the community-dwelling elderly. *Geriatr Gerontol Int.* 2011;11: 267-274.

[14] Jung HW YC, Cho NR, Lee MK, Lee JB. The effect of laughter therapy on sleep in the community-dwelling elderly. *Korean Journal of Family Medicine*. 2009;30: 511-517.

[15] Kim SH, Kook JR, Kwon M, Son MH, Ahn SD, Kim YH. The effects of laughter therapy on mood state and self-esteem in cancer patients undergoing radiation therapy: a randomized controlled trial. *J Altern Complement Med*. 2015;21: 217-222.

[16] Sakai Y, Takayanagi K, Ohno M, Inose R, Fujiwara H. A trial of improvement of immunity in cancer patients by laughter therapy. *Japan-Hospitals*. 2013: 53-59.

[17] Kong M, Shin SH, Lee E, Yun EK. The effect of laughter therapy on radiation dermatitis in patients with breast cancer: a single-blind prospective pilot study. *Onco Targets Ther*. 2014;7: 2053-2059.

[18] Brutsche MH, Grossman P, Muller RE, et al. Impact of laughter on air trapping in severe chronic obstructive lung disease. *Int J Chron Obstruct Pulmon Dis*. 2008;3: 185-192.

[19] Lebowitz KR, Suh S, Diaz PT, Emery CF. Effects of humor and laughter on psychological functioning, quality of life, health status, and pulmonary functioning among patients with chronic obstructive pulmonary disease: a preliminary investigation. Heart and Lung. 2011;40: 310-319.

[20] Hayashi T, Tsujii S, Iburi T, et al. Laughter up-regulates the genes related to NK cell activity in diabetes. Biomed Res. 2007;28: 281-285.

[21] Hayashi T, Urayama O, Hori M, et al. Laughter modulates prorenin receptor gene expression in patients with type 2 diabetes. *J Psychosom Res*. 2007;62: 703-706.

[22] Matsuzaki T, Nakajima A, Ishigami S, Tanno M, Yoshino S. Mirthful laughter differentially affects serum pro- and anti-inflammatory cytokine levels depending on the level of disease activity in patients with rheumatoid arthritis. *Rheumatology* (Oxford). 2006;45: 182-186.

[23] Cho EA, Oh HE. [Effects of laughter therapy on depression, quality of life, resilience and immune responses in breast cancer survivors]. *J Korean Acad Nurs*. 2011;41: 285-293.

EDITOR CONTACT INFORMATION

E. Paul Cherniack, MD
Associate Professor of Clinical Medicine
Department of Medicine Department of Medicine –
Division of Gerontology and Geriatric Medicine
University of Miami Health System, Miami, FL, US
Email: echerniack@med.miami.edu; Evan.Cherniack@va.gov

Tass Holmes, PhD
Anthropology – School of Social and Political Sciences
University of Melbourne, Parkville, Victoria, Australia
Email: tass.holmes@unimelb.edu.au

INDEX

A

B

C

D

E

F

G

H

I

L

M

N

O

P

Q

R

S

T

U

V

W

Y